IØ126177

The Complete Guide to Motivational Interviewing

Interviewing

400 Practical MI Worksheets for Therapists, Counselors, Clinicians and Coaches to Inspire Change and Empower Growth

James Marie Mosley and Willie Candy Shea

Copyright Notice

The Complete Guide to Motivational Interviewing: 400 Practical MI Worksheets for Therapists, Counselors, Clinicians, and Coaches to Inspire Change and Empower Growth
Copyright © 2025 James Marie Mosley and Willie Candy Shea

All rights reserved. No part of this book may be reproduced, distributed, or transmitted in any form or by any means, including photocopying, recording, or other electronic or mechanical methods, without the prior written permission of the authors, except in the case of brief quotations for review purposes or for limited educational and clinical use as outlined below.

This book is intended as a professional resource for therapists, counselors, clinicians, and coaches. While the worksheets and exercises are designed to be **practical tools for use in sessions**, all intellectual property rights remain with the authors.

Guidelines for Reuse of Worksheets

Permitted Use:

- Professionals may **print, photocopy, or digitally share** individual worksheets **for personal clinical use** with clients.

- Educators may **use and distribute** worksheets for teaching and training purposes, provided they do not alter or claim ownership of the material.

- Agencies and institutions may **incorporate worksheets** into programs, training, or therapy sessions, provided proper attribution is given.

Restricted Use:

- Worksheets **may not be resold, compiled into other books, or used for commercial distribution** without explicit written permission from the authors.

- Digital copies of the worksheets **may not be shared online or uploaded to public databases, websites, or forums** without express authorization.

- No modifications or adaptations of the worksheets may be made without prior written consent.

This book is a **tool to support positive change**—please use it **ethically and responsibly** to maintain its integrity and effectiveness.

Disclaimer

This book is not a substitute for professional psychological or medical advice. The exercises are designed to complement therapeutic work but should be used at the discretion of the practitioner. The authors and publishers disclaim any liability for the application of techniques or strategies contained in this book.

First Edition
ISBN: [978-1-7640348-0-7]
Published by: [TherapyBooks Publishing]

Table of Contents

Engaging and Building Rapport 75

Reflective Listening and Communication 209

Strengthening Commitment 403

Maintaining Momentum and Relapse Prevention 453

Preface

Motivational Interviewing (MI) is a powerful approach that helps individuals navigate change, overcome ambivalence, and move toward their goals with confidence. It is built on the foundation of empathy, collaboration, and empowerment—principles that are at the core of every meaningful therapeutic conversation. MI is not about pushing change onto a client but rather drawing out their own motivation, strengths, and commitment.

This book, **The Complete Guide to Motivational Interviewing: 400 Practical MI Worksheets for Therapists, Counselors, Clinicians, and Coaches to Inspire Change and Empower Growth**, was created to serve as a **comprehensive, hands-on resource** for professionals who use MI in their practice. If you are a therapist, counselor, clinician, social worker, or coach, this book will provide you with structured, evidence-based worksheets designed to **enhance your sessions, deepen client engagement, and drive meaningful change**.

Why This Book?

While MI is well-established in the fields of psychotherapy, addiction recovery, healthcare, and coaching, many practitioners struggle with **bridging theory and practice**. They understand MI's core principles but seek practical tools to apply these techniques effectively. This book fills that gap by offering structured worksheets across various **stages of change**, ensuring clients remain engaged, motivated, and committed to their goals.

The worksheets in this book draw from **evidence-based psychological models**, including Self-Determination Theory, Cognitive Behavioral Therapy (CBT), Dialectical Behavior Therapy (DBT), and Positive Psychology. They also incorporate key concepts from pioneers in motivation science, such as **William R. Miller, Stephen Rollnick, Albert Bandura, Carl Rogers, and Edward Deci & Richard Ryan**. These frameworks have been adapted into actionable exercises that guide clients from contemplation to sustained change.

How to Use This Book

This book is divided into **ten core categories**, each addressing different aspects of the change process. The worksheets within these sections are structured to:

- **Explore ambivalence** and resolve conflicting thoughts about change
- **Identify personal values, strengths, and goals**
- **Strengthen commitment and self-efficacy**
- **Develop concrete action plans** that make change realistic
- **Manage setbacks and prevent relapse**
- **Sustain progress and maintain long-term motivation**

Each worksheet follows a consistent format, including a **clear purpose, rationale backed by research, step-by-step instructions, tips for therapists, troubleshooting common challenges, reflection questions, and real-life applications**. This structured approach ensures that each tool is **effective, user-friendly, and immediately applicable in session**.

Who Is This Book For?

This book is designed for **any professional working in behavior change**:

- **Therapists, psychologists, and counselors** working in mental health, addiction treatment, and personal development
- **Social workers and case managers** helping clients transition through life's challenges
- **Health and wellness coaches** supporting clients with fitness, nutrition, and self-care goals
- **Educators and career coaches** assisting students or professionals in making informed decisions
- **Medical professionals** guiding patients through chronic illness management or lifestyle changes

Whether you are new to MI or an experienced practitioner, this book will provide **ready-to-use worksheets** that simplify complex concepts and help you implement MI strategies effectively.

A Final Thought

Change is not always easy, but the right support can make all the difference. **Motivational Interviewing empowers people to tap into their strengths, build confidence, and take control of their own transformation**. As you use this book, I encourage you to **bring your own warmth, curiosity, and authenticity to the**

process. No worksheet can replace the power of genuine human connection, but together, they can create a structured, compassionate, and empowering experience for every client.

Thank you for your commitment to guiding others toward meaningful change. Let's begin.

Introduction

Motivational Interviewing (MI) is a collaborative approach that helps clients find their own reasons for change. By focusing on open-ended questions, reflective listening, and empathy, therapists and counselors can assist individuals in discovering solutions that emerge from their unique perspectives and experiences. **This book provides 400 worksheets and exercises** spanning the core processes of MI—engaging, focusing, evoking, and planning—while integrating additional skills such as reflective listening, rolling with resistance, and developing discrepancy. All these worksheets are designed with flexibility in mind, enabling professionals from **diverse fields**—mental health, healthcare, social work, education, coaching, and beyond—to adopt these strategies effectively.

The Heart of MI

MI respects the autonomy of clients and emphasizes the importance of eliciting change talk from within rather than imposing external directives. This method hinges on a few key principles:

1. **Express Empathy**

   o Therapists show genuine understanding of a client's viewpoint.

   o Judgments are kept at bay, and non-verbal cues support an atmosphere of trust.

2. **Develop Discrepancy**

   o Clients reflect on how their current behaviors might clash with their deeper values or goals.

   o Heightening awareness of this gap can fuel motivation to explore and implement new actions.

3. **Roll with Resistance**

   o Rather than confronting or arguing, therapists maintain a stance of curiosity and openness.

- Clients' hesitancies or objections become opportunities for further exploration.

4. **Support Self-Efficacy**

   - The therapist focuses on the client's strengths and past successes.

   - Each step toward positive behavior change is celebrated to reinforce confidence.

The Structure of This Resource

This collection of 400 worksheets is organized into **ten categories**, each reflecting an important theme in MI:

1. **Foundational Exercises** (40 worksheets)

2. **Engaging and Building Rapport** (40 worksheets)

3. **Focusing and Setting the Agenda** (40 worksheets)

4. **Evoking Change Talk** (40 worksheets)

5. **Reflective Listening and Communication** (40 worksheets)

6. **Rolling with Resistance** (40 worksheets)

7. **Developing Discrepancy** (40 worksheets)

8. **Goal Setting and Planning** (40 worksheets)

9. **Strengthening Commitment** (40 worksheets)

10. **Maintaining Momentum and Relapse Prevention** (40 worksheets)

Each category begins with a brief overview, followed by worksheets specifically tailored to strengthen the corresponding MI skill. The intention is to provide adaptable tools for **all professions** that employ motivational interviewing techniques, whether you are a clinician in a hospital, a social worker in a community center, or a life coach supporting personal growth.

Why Worksheets?

Clarity: Worksheets give structure. They let clients put abstract thoughts onto paper, making those ideas more concrete and actionable.

Ownership: When clients write their own pros, cons, and goals, they see their own language staring back at them. This sense of ownership often sparks genuine commitment.

Depth: A simple "Pros and Cons" worksheet can reveal deeper fears or hopes. A "Values Mapping" sheet might expose how a client's core beliefs line up with their goals. Such realizations boost motivation and reduce confusion.

Progress Tracking: Worksheets turn one-time insights into lasting records. Clients can revisit them, notice patterns, and feel encouraged by visible progress.

Example:
A client struggling with alcohol use might fill out a "Reasons to Change" worksheet. At first, they list typical items like health or finances. But as they go deeper—without the therapist telling them "You must do this"—they might discover an emotional reason: wanting to be a better role model for their kids. Reading their own words, they often think, "That's it. That's why I need to cut back." This reflection, captured on paper, fuels determination and keeps them anchored through harder days.

In essence, **MI worksheets** blend conversation with tangible actions. They let therapists keep sessions focused while allowing clients to see their motivations laid out plainly. This dual approach—talk plus written reflection—drives meaningful change.

How to use the worksheets

Motivational Interviewing (MI) worksheets can serve as practical tools that guide both you and your client through the key stages of change. They are typically grouped into categories—Engaging and Building Rapport, Focusing and Setting the Agenda, Evoking Change Talk, Strengthening Commitment, and Maintaining Momentum and Relapse Prevention. Each category zeroes in on a specific MI process: from establishing rapport to identifying the client's values, eliciting their own reasons for change, making clear plans, and finally preventing relapse.

To begin, it is vital to choose worksheets that match the client's stage or needs. For instance, if they are unsure about therapy or reluctant to talk, rapport-building sheets help you understand their interests and shape a safe environment. At this early phase, worksheets on active listening or warmth can set a tone of respect and collaboration. Next, the focusing sheets help both parties define and sharpen the main goals—like clarifying a client's priorities or laying out a workable target. This ensures you are aligned on what the client truly wants to address.

Once the direction is set, you use evoking worksheets to uncover the client's deeper motivations. Worksheets that prompt them to name their desire, ability, reasons, and need for change encourage stronger self-motivation. These exercises highlight the client's intrinsic capacity rather than imposing external advice. If they start voicing genuine commitment, you progress to commitment worksheets that fortify their resolve—like drafting a statement of dedication or identifying daily habits that keep them moving forward.

Throughout, it is helpful to incorporate accountability elements: maintenance and relapse-prevention worksheets. These can include logs or checklists to record progress, a designated accountability partner, or crisis plans that guide the client when they sense a backslide coming. The idea is to blend reflection (why change matters) with concrete action (exact tasks, next steps, or alternative coping strategies).

In session, you can pull up a relevant worksheet and walk the client through each section, encouraging them to fill in answers. Then, you discuss the responses, highlighting their own strengths. Between sessions, they can keep using these sheets to note triggers, track small wins, or manage setbacks. By systematically combining reflection, planning, and review, the worksheets help the client take manageable steps while retaining autonomy, ensuring MI remains a collaborative, empathic, and client-driven process.

Below are some scenarios to demonstrate how these worksheets can be implemented in your practice.

Scenario One: Managing Work Stress and Preventing Burnout

James, 34, is an enthusiastic project manager at a bustling software firm. Over the past year, he has taken on extra tasks, hoping to impress his bosses. Lately, he feels chronically exhausted, snapping at colleagues and sleeping poorly. He realises he might be heading toward burnout but fears cutting back might ruin his image at work. He decides to explore Motivational Interviewing (MI) techniques and relevant worksheets to restore balance, lower stress, and keep his career moving positively.

James's therapist begins with worksheets from the **Engaging and Building Rapport** category. She first uses **Worksheet #2: "Client Interests Exploration" (Engaging and Building Rapport)** to learn more about his favourite hobbies and what he finds meaningful outside of work. James admits it has been months since he played guitar or saw friends. He notices how stress has pushed aside his personal life. Feeling heard and understood, he relaxes in therapy, willing to define a new approach.

They move next to the **Focusing and Setting the Agenda** category, picking **Worksheet #1: "Goal Brainstorm" (Focusing and Setting the Agenda).** James lists possible aims: limiting overtime, scheduling leisure time, delegating tasks, or learning to say no. Together, they refine a single overarching goal: "Reduce weekly work hours from 60 to about 45 while still maintaining quality performance." This aim speaks to James's desire for healthier boundaries without quitting his job.

To deepen motivation, they turn to the **Evoking Change Talk** category with **Worksheet #4: "Change Talk Brainstorm" (Evoking Change Talk).** James outlines reasons for change: better mental health, improved sleep, and returning to guitar practice. The therapist reflects his statements: "It sounds like you really miss that creative outlet and feel disappointed that your free time vanished." Hearing his own reasons amplified helps James see he can reclaim both productivity and well-being.

They also consult the **Strengthening Commitment** category. Using **Worksheet #7: "Commitment Statement" (Strengthening Commitment),** James composes:
"I commit to balancing my workload and personal life because I want long-term health and wish to remain an energetic leader at the company."
He keeps this statement on a sticky note at his desk as a reminder whenever he feels the urge to pile on extra tasks.

Identifying Stress Triggers and Barriers

Next, James clarifies his main triggers for burnout. They consult **Worksheet #2: "Relapse Risk Factors" (Maintaining Momentum and Relapse Prevention).** James sees typical triggers:

- Multiple urgent deadlines hitting at once.

- Fear of disappointing superiors, prompting him to say "yes" to every request.

- Anxiety at night that leads him to check emails instead of sleeping.

He realises that ignoring these triggers has steadily eroded his energy. The therapist helps him adapt the plan to manage each risk. For urgent deadlines, James decides to prioritise two or three tasks daily, leaving smaller ones for the team. For fear of disapproval, he plans to have honest chats with management about realistic timelines. For nighttime email-checking, he sets a cut-off of 9 p.m., enabling him to wind down.

They also use **Worksheet #5: "Early Warning System" (Maintaining Momentum and Relapse Prevention).** James notes early signs he's sliding into unhealthy patterns: skipping lunch, snapping at coworkers, or feeling dread on Sunday nights. He commits to noticing these signals and reacting quickly—perhaps by scheduling half an hour offline midday or taking a short walk to clear his head before it spirals.

Creating a Realistic Action Plan

With these triggers in mind, they draft a strategy using **Worksheet #3: "Action Step Breakdown" (Focusing and Setting the Agenda).** Each step includes:

1. **Morning Checklist**: He'll map top priorities for the day, ensuring no more than three major tasks.

2. **Afternoon Recharge**: He'll block 15 minutes after lunch to step outside or practise quick guitar exercises on a pocket app.

3. **Delegation**: Once a week, he'll identify tasks someone else can handle, giving teammates new responsibilities.

4. **No-Work Evenings**: After 9 p.m., he'll avoid emails, using that time to relax or sleep.

6

James tests feasibility with **Worksheet #4: "Plan Feasibility Check" (Focusing and Setting the Agenda).** He notices potential obstacles: some tasks might feel too critical to delegate. His therapist suggests partial delegation or open conversation with his boss about distributing tasks fairly. James sees it's doable if he clarifies job roles with management.

Building Accountability and Tracking Progress

To maintain momentum, James picks a friend at the office to serve as an accountability partner, referencing **Worksheet #6: "Accountability Structure" (Strengthening Commitment).** They decide on quick Friday check-ins: Did James keep to 45-hour weeks? Did he practise self-care? Knowing someone else expects these updates encourages him to stay aligned with his plan.

Additionally, they incorporate **Worksheet #3: "Maintenance Checklist" (Maintaining Momentum and Relapse Prevention).** James sets daily or weekly tasks:

- Tick if he limited daily hours to about 8 or 9.

- Note if he delegated at least one item.

- Write short reflections on how free time felt.

This structured routine helps James track improvements. After two weeks, he finds that simply logging daily hours makes him question whether that extra hour is truly necessary.

Navigating Setbacks and Building Self-Compassion

Two months in, James experiences a crunch period—three big client projects land simultaneously. He reverts to 60-hour weeks for a bit. Angry at himself, he returns to therapy feeling defeated. The therapist suggests **Worksheet #8: "Turning Setbacks into Lessons" (Strengthening Commitment).** James analyses:

- The cause: sudden client demands, limited staff.

- The mistake: not pushing back or asking for help early.

- The lesson: next time, open a dialogue with his boss about realistic deadlines.

Using **Worksheet #10: "Self-Compassion During Slips" (Maintaining Momentum and Relapse Prevention),** James realises blaming himself harshly only worsens stress. He writes kinder statements: "This slip doesn't define me. I can adjust strategies and do better tomorrow." The gentler approach restores hope and motivation.

Maintaining Long-Term Balance

Finally, they shape a long-term relapse prevention plan. James uses **Worksheet #9: "Detecting Complacency" (Maintaining Momentum and Relapse Prevention).** If he finds he's ignoring lunch or ignoring daily planning, that's a red flag. He vows to correct course quickly. He also sets a monthly "Progress Audit," referencing **Worksheet #5: "Regular Progress Audits" (Maintaining Momentum).** Each month, he reviews total hours worked, stress levels, and guitar practice frequency. If the numbers climb or he's skipping personal breaks, he'll revisit the worksheets, check triggers, and refine solutions.

James invests in a few new personal goals, perhaps scheduling a guitar lesson or joining a weekend jam group. The sense of a fulfilling life outside the office cements his commitment to healthy boundaries. He sees that "burnout prevention" is not just about working less but also about energising himself with meaningful pursuits.

Conclusion of Scenario

Through combining multiple MI worksheets—each belonging to a relevant category—James moves from overwork and chronic stress toward a sustainable, healthy routine. The "Engaging and Building Rapport" set fosters trust and openness, "Focusing and Setting the Agenda" clarifies his aims and steps, "Evoking Change Talk" galvanises his internal motivations, "Strengthening Commitment" keeps him determined even after stumbles, and "Maintaining Momentum and Relapse Prevention" provides a vigilant framework. Over time, James reclaims control over his work schedule and invests in a balanced lifestyle, significantly reducing his risk of burnout. As he sees real progress in both job performance and personal well-being, James feels proud that he can serve his company effectively without sacrificing his health—a win-win anchored in consistent self-awareness and strategic action.

Scenario Two: Recovering from Emotional Eating and Building Healthy Relationships with Food

Simone is 29 and struggles with emotional eating whenever she feels anxious or lonely. She has tried restrictive diets, only to end up binging on sweets late at night. Tired of yo-yo patterns and guilt, she seeks help using Motivational Interviewing, hoping to form kinder, lasting habits around food and stress management.

Simone's therapist first turns to **Worksheet #1: "Warm Connections" (Engaging and Building Rapport)** in the Engaging and Building Rapport category. She invites Simone to talk about her daily life, favourite activities, and the role food plays beyond just nutrition. Simone realises that certain triggers—like stressful emails from her boss or late-night loneliness—prompt her to seek comfort in sugary treats.

They move on to "Focusing and Setting the Agenda." Simone completes **Worksheet #2: "Goal Brainstorm" (Focusing and Setting the Agenda)**: potential objectives include controlling nighttime snacking, cooking balanced meals, or finding alternative ways to handle stress. She refines a main goal: "Reduce emotional eating episodes to once a week or less, replacing them with healthy coping or planned snacks."

Evoking Real Motivation for Change

Using **Worksheet #3: "Change Talk Brainstorm" (Evoking Change Talk)** from the Evoking Change Talk category, Simone pinpoints:

- **Desire**: "I want to feel more in control around food."

- **Ability**: "I can cook well and enjoy fresh meals if I plan."

- **Reasons**: "Binges leave me bloated, self-critical, and disconnected from social events."

- **Need**: "My mental health suffers when I see the cycle repeating."

Hearing Simone's statements, the therapist reflects: "You sound genuinely eager to break the guilt and embarrassment." Simone, seeing her reasons validated, feels ready to progress.

Strengthening Commitment

They move to the Strengthening Commitment category. **Worksheet #7: "Commitment Statement" (Strengthening Commitment)** helps Simone write: "I commit to managing my emotions without turning to food as my primary outlet because I deserve mental peace and a healthier body."
She keeps this statement in her kitchen, a visible reminder that her choice stems from self-respect rather than punishment.

She also tries **Worksheet #8: "Barrier-Busting Mindset" (Strengthening Commitment).** She lists typical mental barriers: "I deserve a treat after a bad day," or "One snack won't hurt." Then she crafts counters, like "I deserve kindness, not temporary sugar spikes." Rehearsing these affirmations prepares her for tough moments.

Designing a Practical Plan Around Eating

Using **Worksheet #3: "Action Step Breakdown" (Focusing and Setting the Agenda)**, Simone details:

1. Plan balanced meals each Sunday, including some sweet but moderate dessert to avoid feeling deprived.

2. Identify a short list of alternative activities for emotional spikes—like journalling, quick yoga, or texting a friend.

3. Keep a daily log of triggers, emotions, and whether she used a coping tool or ended up snacking.

She checks feasibility with **Worksheet #4: "Plan Feasibility Check" (Focusing).** Simone realises she might skip meal prep if she's exhausted. So she commits to simpler recipes or batch cooking. If she faces strong evening cravings, she might allow a portion-controlled treat but practise mindful eating.

Mindful Awareness and Emotional Coping

Simone references the **Maintaining Momentum and Relapse Prevention** category, starting with **Worksheet #2: "Relapse Risk Factors."** She sees triggers:

- Post-work anxiety.

- Feeling lonely on Friday nights if friends are busy.

- High stress from her father's recent health scare.

She pairs each with a coping strategy. For anxiety after work, she'll do a 10-minute wind-down routine before dinner. For loneliness, she might schedule a phone call or plan an at-home spa session. For bigger stress, she might speak to a sibling for emotional support or consider therapy if it worsens.

She also uses **Worksheet #5: "Early Warning System" (Maintaining Momentum).** Simone notes subtle signs like daydreaming about pastries or telling herself "I deserve an entire box of donuts." When she sees these thoughts, she'll do a short breathing exercise or text a friend. The small pause helps her pivot away from impulsive snacking.

Accountability and Logging Progress

Simone picks a friend from her gym class as an accountability partner, referencing **Worksheet #6: "Accountability Structure" (Strengthening Commitment).** They agree on brief nightly messages: "How did your day go? Any binge urge?" This open dialogue keeps Simone mindful of her emotional state.

She also keeps a **Maintenance Checklist** (Maintaining Momentum). Each day, she ticks off:

- **Meal planning** done or not.

- **Any emotional spikes** and which coping method used.

- **Total sweets consumed** or any unplanned binge.

Celebrating small victories is crucial. Using **Worksheet #9: "Celebrating Small Victories" (Strengthening Commitment),** Simone might treat herself with a relaxing bath or a new eBook if she completes a binge-free week. Each mini celebration boosts her confidence in the new path.

Navigating Setbacks

Sure enough, Simone experiences a slip after a distressing call regarding her father's health. She impulsively devours a tub of ice cream. She revisits **Worksheet #8: "Turning Setbacks into Lessons" (Strengthening Commitment)**:

- **Trigger**: Emotional turmoil.

- **Lesson**: In intense family stress, she needs bigger emotional support or therapy check-ins.

- **Forward step**: She decides to store single-portion ice creams or keep healthier sweet options. She also calls her brother more often to share updates.

The therapist encourages **Worksheet #10: "Self-Compassion During Slips" (Maintaining Momentum).** Simone writes gentle self-talk: "It's okay to be upset. One slip doesn't negate progress." Freed from excessive guilt, she realises she can keep going.

Reviewing Gains and Sustaining Growth

After a few months, Simone finds her binges dropped significantly. She references **Worksheet #4: "Reviewing Successes" (Maintaining Momentum)**:

- She has fewer sugar-fueled nights, replaced with journalling or short yoga.

- She's discovered new snack recipes that feel satisfying but not excessive.

- She's more aware of her emotions, noticing stress sooner and acting kindly.

Her weight has stabilised somewhat, but more importantly, her mood is calmer. She finalises with **Worksheet #3: "Final Reflection" (Maintaining Momentum).** She sees how MI-based worksheets guided her from feeling powerless around food to building an emotionally healthy relationship with eating. She now recognises each day is a chance to practise mindful choices, with slip-ups as learning moments, not moral failings.

In conclusion, Simone's success stems from systematically using Engaging worksheets to reveal her triggers, Focusing worksheets to set feasible steps, Evoking worksheets to anchor her inner reasons, Strengthening Commitment to maintain resolve, and Maintaining Momentum to handle real-life obstacles. Through consistent self-awareness, planning, and a supportive accountability system, Simone transforms emotional eating into a balanced, self-compassionate approach to food and stress.

Scenario Three: Supporting a Teen's Motivation to Stay in School and Manage Peer Pressure

Marie is a 16-year-old student who has started skipping classes, feeling that school is pointless. She's drawn to a group of friends who likewise dismiss academic goals. Marie's parents and teachers are concerned. She reluctantly agrees to Motivational Interviewing (MI) sessions to see if she can rekindle interest in her education. The therapist uses several MI worksheets from different categories—**Engaging and Building Rapport**, **Focusing and Setting the Agenda**, **Evoking Change Talk**, **Strengthening Commitment**, and **Maintaining Momentum and Relapse Prevention**—to help Marie find intrinsic reasons to stay in school and resist negative peer pressure.

Marie's therapist first uses **Worksheet #3: "Cultural and Contextual Inquiry" (Engaging and Building Rapport)**. They talk about Marie's background: she's bored with classes, craving acceptance from peers who label school as dull. She confesses she doesn't relate to her parents' old-fashioned expectations. The therapist acknowledges her need to feel understood, building trust.

They shift to **Worksheet #1: "Goal Brainstorm" (Focusing and Setting the Agenda)**. Marie lists possible aims:

- Attending classes more consistently.

- Passing this semester without massive stress.

- Possibly exploring an after-school club or activity that suits her.
  She decides the main focus is: "Attend at least 90% of my classes this term and explore one extracurricular interest."

Exploring Deeper Motivation

To flesh out her reasons, the therapist employs **Worksheet #2: "Evoking from Ambivalence" (Evoking Change Talk)**. Marie sees she's torn: part of her wants to fit

13

in with friends, while another side recognises that dropping grades threaten future opportunities. She identifies the following:

- **Desire**: She wants to graduate without feeling trapped in summer school.

- **Ability**: She's passed classes before when she put in effort.

- **Reasons**: She dreams of eventually living independently, needing some formal credentials.

- **Need**: She can't keep lying to her parents about truancy; it's causing tension at home.

Hearing her own arguments, Marie feels a spark of motivation. The therapist reflects: "It sounds like you do see a real point in finishing school, even if your friends mock it." Marie nods, admitting she's tired of the stress. She then completes **Worksheet #7: "Commitment Statement" (Strengthening Commitment)**:
"I commit to showing up for classes and discovering something at school I can enjoy, because I want a real future and to feel proud of myself."

Laying Out a Concrete Path

They then use **Worksheet #3: "Action Step Breakdown" (Focusing and Setting the Agenda).** Marie shapes small steps:

1. **Nightly Prep**: Laying out clothes and supplies so she's less tempted to skip in the morning.

2. **Attendance Tracker**: Marking each successful day of full attendance on a phone calendar.

3. **Explore One Club**: Checking out a drama or art club within two weeks.

They check feasibility via **Worksheet #4: "Plan Feasibility Check" (Focusing and Setting the Agenda).** Marie worries her friends will pressure her to ditch. She decides if they push her, she'll say she must raise grades or her parents will ground her (a partial truth). The therapist encourages her to stand by her personal reasons too, but using a practical excuse might help in the moment.

Balancing Peer Influence

14

Marie tries **Worksheet #6: "Boundaries to Protect Change" (Strengthening Commitment).** She identifies that skipping becomes likely if certain friends text her early to hang out at a café instead of school. She plans to silence her phone during mornings, reactivating it after she's on campus. She also sets a boundary: if they're urging her to skip more than once, she'll politely decline and walk away.

She references **Worksheet #2: "Relapse Risk Factors" (Maintaining Momentum and Relapse Prevention).** Potential pitfalls:

- Feeling "too cool" to attend a dull class.

- Last-minute texts from friends offering something more fun.

- Accumulated fatigue from staying up late on her phone.

She builds responses like going to bed earlier and ignoring morning invites. If boredom in class hits, she'll doodle or write quietly instead of fleeing.

Encouraging Consistency and Reflecting on Progress

To stay accountable, Marie uses **Worksheet #3: "Maintenance Checklist" (Maintaining Momentum and Relapse Prevention).** Each school day, she notes:

- Did she attend all classes?

- Did she attempt to participate or at least stay engaged?

- How did she handle peer pressure?

At the end of each week, the therapist encourages a brief review with **Worksheet #4: "Reviewing Successes" (Maintaining Momentum and Relapse Prevention).** They highlight any days she overcame the temptation to skip, or a new conversation she had with classmates who aren't part of her old crowd. Celebrating small wins fosters her sense of capability. For instance, she might treat herself to a new art supply if she completes two weeks of perfect attendance.

Overcoming Hurdles and Using Self-Compassion

A few weeks in, Marie slips. She oversleeps and skips an entire day, meeting up with her friends. She dreads telling her therapist. However, they use **Worksheet #8: "Turning Setbacks into Lessons" (Strengthening Commitment).** She realises:

- Trigger: She felt tired and unmotivated that morning, then saw a group chat invitation.

- Lesson: She can set an earlier bedtime, plus charge her phone away from her bed. If an invite arrives, she ignores it until after school.

She references **Worksheet #10: "Self-Compassion During Slips" (Maintaining Momentum and Relapse Prevention).** Instead of calling herself a "failure," she writes a gentler note: "I messed up one day, but I'm still committed. Tomorrow is a fresh start." This perspective keeps her from spiraling into giving up entirely.

Finding Internal Rewards

Because motivation can't solely be about avoiding punishment, the therapist revisits **Worksheet #1: "Feeling the Benefits" (Strengthening Commitment).** Marie identifies internal positives from attending class:

- She's less anxious about lying to parents.

- She can keep up with assignments, reducing last-minute stress.

- She might discover new interests or at least maintain future college options.

Each time she acknowledges these benefits, it reinforces that the small daily choice to attend class has real payoffs. She also tries an extracurricular club. To her surprise, she connects with a group of students who share an interest in painting murals. That sense of belonging outside her old circle elevates her confidence.

Sustaining Momentum and Identity Shifts

To prevent relapse long-term, Marie checks **Worksheet #9: "Detecting Complacency" (Maintaining Momentum and Relapse Prevention).** If she notices feeling "It's fine to skip again—no big deal," she'll read her commitment statement or recall how stressful it was lying at home. Regular accountability with her new art club peers also helps; if she doesn't show up, they'll wonder where she is.

She shifts her self-view with **Worksheet #5: "Shifting Identity" (Maintaining Momentum and Relapse Prevention).** Instead of seeing herself as "someone bored by school," she now thinks: "I'm a creative student exploring new opportunities." This identity shift nudges her to keep an open mind. Over time, she aligns more with activities that feed her interests.

Final Reflection

After a few months, Marie's attendance is at 90%. She's improved in a couple of subjects and feels less reliant on rebellious peers to feel cool. She completes **Worksheet #3: "Final Reflection" (Maintaining Momentum and Relapse Prevention).** She notes:

- **Before**: She felt no point in classes and let peer pressure shape her days.

- **Now**: She mostly attends, sees glimpses of personal growth, and discovered an art group that she actually enjoys.

- **Ongoing plan**: Keep morning phone boundaries, maintain contact with supportive friends, remain watchful of urges to skip when a class feels boring.

From being on the verge of dropping out, Marie transitions to an active, if still somewhat cautious, student who believes in finishing school. She sees these changes formed by applying MI worksheets systematically—identifying triggers, clarifying personal values, building resilience against peer pressure, and nurturing a sense of autonomy. Through consistent reflection and small, tangible steps, she grows confident that she can chart her own path rather than blindly follow her friends' negativity.

Scenario Four: Managing Chronic Health Conditions with Self-Care

Paula is 50, newly diagnosed with type 2 diabetes. She feels overwhelmed by numerous instructions—modify her diet, exercise regularly, track blood sugar, keep doctor appointments. She's used to a leisurely lifestyle and comfort foods, and these changes feel daunting. Paula realises her health is at stake but struggles to break old habits. She seeks Motivational Interviewing (MI) to build a realistic plan for better self-care, hoping to avoid long-term complications.

Building Rapport and Clarifying Objectives

In the initial session, Paula's therapist engages her using **Worksheet #2: "Client Interests Exploration" (Engaging and Building Rapport)**. They discuss Paula's routine: she enjoys watching TV after work, doesn't like structured exercise, and occasionally bakes sugary treats. She admits, "I know it's not good for my diabetes, but it's how I unwind." The therapist empathises, noting that these comforts are hard to give up overnight.

They move to **Worksheet #1: "Goal Brainstorm" (Focusing and Setting the Agenda)**, where Paula lists possible aims:

- Reducing sugary snacks.

- Doing some mild exercise, at least walking.

- Taking medication consistently.

- Monitoring her blood sugar daily.

They refine it into a single overarching objective: "Implement a manageable daily self-care routine that supports stable blood sugar and overall health." Paula wants to avoid extremes and set small steps that feel sustainable.

Eliciting Reasons for Change and Strengthening Motivation

The therapist guides Paula to reflect on her deeper motivations using **Worksheet #3: "Change Talk Brainstorm" (Evoking Change Talk)**. Paula identifies:

- **Desire**: "I want to feel more energetic, not so sluggish in the afternoons."

- **Ability**: "I've followed meal plans before when I tried dieting, so I know I can do it in increments."

- **Reasons**: "I'm worried about future complications, like nerve issues or heart problems."

- **Need**: "I need to manage stress in better ways than just eating sweets."

18

They write these reasons on a note Paula keeps in her kitchen. She sees that caring for herself aligns with her long-term well-being and the wish to stay active for her grandchildren. To solidify, Paula completes **Worksheet #7: "Commitment Statement" (Strengthening Commitment)**: "I commit to consistent self-care for my diabetes because I value a long, healthy life and want to be active with my family."

Crafting a Practical Self-Care Plan

Using **Worksheet #3: "Action Step Breakdown" (Focusing and Setting the Agenda)**, Paula and her therapist chart small, concrete tasks:

1. **Diet Adjustments**:

    o Replace sugary desserts on weekdays with fresh fruit or sugar-free options.

    o Start each week by planning a simple menu, focusing on balanced meals recommended by her dietitian.

2. **Physical Activity**:

    o Begin daily 15-minute walks after dinner.

    o On weekends, try a gentle 30-minute indoor dance routine or stretching video.

3. **Medication and Monitoring**:

    o Take prescribed medication at set times (morning and evening).

    o Check blood sugar each morning and log it in a notebook.

They test feasibility with **Worksheet #4: "Plan Feasibility Check" (Focusing)**. Paula foresees challenges: possible sweet cravings after stressful days, sometimes too tired to walk. They decide she can skip a walk if fatigue is too high, but she must do a 5-minute stretching session instead, preventing a total break from movement.

Identifying Triggers and Stress Points

Paula references **Worksheet #2: "Relapse Risk Factors" (Maintaining Momentum and Relapse Prevention)** for her diabetes management context. She sees triggers for unhealthy eating:

- Emotional stress after tough workdays.

- Family gatherings with rich desserts.

- Late-night TV watching, which triggers snacking urges.

She outlines coping methods for each risk factor. For stress, she might do a quick breathing exercise. For family gatherings, bring a healthier dessert alternative or eat a satisfying meal beforehand. For late-night snacking, schedule a short phone call with a supportive friend or read a relaxing book instead of focusing on food.

She also uses **Worksheet #5: "Early Warning System" (Maintaining Momentum and Relapse Prevention).** She jots down subtle signals like "feeling anxious around 9 p.m." or "persistent thoughts of sugary comfort foods." Once she notices those signs, she can quickly pivot to a chosen coping tactic (fruit, herbal tea, or a short walk in place).

Accountability and Tracking

To foster consistency, Paula pairs up with a coworker who also aims for healthier habits. They review **Worksheet #6: "Accountability Structure" (Strengthening Commitment).** They decide on brief weekly chats, asking, "How's your meal planning or sugar monitoring going?" Paula also commits to **Worksheet #3: "Maintenance Checklist" (Maintaining Momentum)**:

- **Daily**:

    - Mark if she followed a planned breakfast-lunch-dinner outline.

    - Note if she did a 15-minute walk or alternative activity.

    - Record blood sugar in her log.

- **Weekly**:

- Evaluate if she met her goals most days. If not, see which strategy to refine.

By visually tracking these tasks, Paula quickly sees patterns. For instance, if she misses walks on days she works late, she might plan a brief midday walk or an earlier dinner to free up time.

Handling Slips and Encouraging Self-Kindness

After a month, Paula experiences a slip during a stressful project at work. She ends up eating an entire box of cookies over two evenings. She feels guilty, worrying that she's undone her progress. The therapist introduces **Worksheet #8: "Turning Setbacks into Lessons" (Strengthening Commitment).** Paula realises:

- **Trigger**: She felt overwhelmed, didn't plan her meals that week.

- **Lesson**: She can carve out 10 minutes on Sunday nights for meal prep, even if busy.

- **Adjustment**: She'll keep a small stash of healthy snacks at the office to avoid extreme cravings.

They also practise **Worksheet #10: "Self-Compassion During Slips" (Maintaining Momentum).** Paula writes a statement: "One rough week doesn't erase my efforts. I'll restart meal planning and reaffirm my reasons for better health." This gentler mindset prevents a downward spiral of shame.

Monitoring Improvements and Evolving Goals

Paula's short walks become more enjoyable. She occasionally extends them to 25 minutes if she feels good. She notices her blood sugar readings are stabilising. Using **Worksheet #4: "Reviewing Successes" (Maintaining Momentum),** she highlights:

- She's halved her dessert intake.

- She's more consistent with medication times.

- She feels lighter and more energetic at work.

She decides to fine-tune her goals using **Worksheet #9: "Flexible Goal Updates" (Maintaining Momentum).** Maybe she'll aim for two 20-minute walks daily or try a gentle yoga class on weekends. This evolution keeps her engaged, preventing boredom with the routine.

Guarding Against Complacency and Long-Term Relapse

Paula references **Worksheet #5: "Detecting Complacency" (Maintaining Momentum).** If she finds herself skipping blood sugar checks or ignoring portion sizes because "Everything's fine now," that's a warning sign. She commits to monthly progress audits to confirm her regimen is stable.

She keeps an "Emergency Contact Sheet" with a friend or diabetes educator if she experiences emotional or medical crises. She also sets a "Checklist for Crisis" if her blood sugar spikes or if stress triggers her old binge patterns. Immediate steps might include calling a friend, taking medication as prescribed, or scheduling an urgent doctor's consult if needed.

Final Reflection and Outlook

After several months, Paula sees meaningful improvements: she's lost some weight healthily, her blood sugar is more manageable, and she's feeling more confident. She tries **Worksheet #3: "Final Reflection" (Maintaining Momentum).** She writes:

- **Before**: She felt daunted by diabetes care, seeking sugary solace under stress.

- **Now**: She follows a balanced meal plan, exercises moderately, and acknowledges slip-ups as part of learning.

- **Lessons**: Tiny daily actions—like a short walk or meal prep—accumulate to big health benefits.

- **Future**: She's open to exploring new hobbies (like a light dance class) to keep her routine fresh.

Paula remains vigilant, understanding that type 2 diabetes is a chronic condition needing ongoing management. But MI worksheets offered a roadmap from initial reluctance to taking purposeful, life-affirming steps. By weaving together reflection on values, structured planning, accountability, and a self-compassionate stance, Paula has built a foundation for lasting health improvements.

Scenario Five: Finding New Career Direction After Layoff

Gianni is 42 and was recently laid off from a manufacturing firm that downsized. He's spent 15 years in the same type of role and now feels disoriented. Should he look for a similar position or explore a whole new path? He's overwhelmed by the thought of rejections and uncertain about retraining. Afraid of making the wrong move, he's delaying any job search. By using Motivational Interviewing (MI) worksheets, Gianni hopes to clarify his professional goals, revive self-confidence, and break free from this paralysis.

Building Rapport and Determining Focus

Gianni's therapist begins with **Worksheet #1: "Warm Connections" (Engaging and Building Rapport)** to create a trusting environment. Gianni reveals he once loved tinkering with machinery, but his previous job grew routine. He's also a devoted cyclist on weekends. The therapist notes his practical side and how he finds satisfaction in hands-on activities.

They move on to **Worksheet #1: "Goal Brainstorm" (Focusing and Setting the Agenda).** Gianni lists potential objectives:

- Seek a similar manufacturing role.

- Explore a complete career pivot (bike shop technician, mechanical design, or something else).

- Return to school or get certifications.

They settle on a main goal: "Identify and pursue at least two promising career paths within the next two months, applying for relevant positions or training programs."

Exploring Internal Motivations

They use **Worksheet #3: "Change Talk Brainstorm" (Evoking Change Talk)** to unearth Gianni's reasons for re-entering the workforce with clarity:

- **Desire**: "I want to wake up feeling excited about my work again."

- **Ability**: "I've honed mechanical skills and have experience leading small teams."

- **Reasons**: "I need to support my family's finances and restore my sense of purpose."

- **Need**: "Sitting idle is eroding my confidence."

Hearing these statements reflected back, Gianni grows more convinced he can try new routes. He also completes **Worksheet #7: "Commitment Statement" (Strengthening Commitment)**:

"I commit to exploring new career opportunities and applying to them because I want a fulfilling future and refuse to let this layoff define me."

Forming a Concrete Plan

Next, they employ **Worksheet #3: "Action Step Breakdown" (Focusing and Setting the Agenda)**:

1. **Self-Assessment**: Spend a week mapping out Gianni's key skills, including mechanical know-how, leadership, and problem-solving.

2. **Industry Research**: Investigate at least three job fields (traditional manufacturing, local bike shops, mechanical design roles).

3. **Training or Certification Inquiry**: Spend an afternoon contacting technical schools or online programs about short courses.

4. **Application and Networking**: Update résumé, apply to at least two job postings, and reach out to old colleagues for potential leads.

They do **Worksheet #4: "Plan Feasibility Check" (Focusing and Setting the Agenda).** Gianni worries about rejection. The therapist points out smaller first steps— like contacting a community college about evening courses—might help him gauge what's viable. If he feels hesitant about applying for advanced design roles, he can start with something slightly less intimidating, like reaching out to a local bike repair store to shadow a technician.

Identifying Triggers and Self-Doubt

Gianni references **Worksheet #2: "Relapse Risk Factors" (Maintaining Momentum and Relapse Prevention)**, focusing on what might derail his job search:

- Memories of past rejection letters.

- Anxiety about new technology he's unfamiliar with.

- Pressure from family who might be anxious about finances.

He outlines coping strategies. For rejection letters, he decides to store them in a folder and remind himself they're part of the process, not a personal condemnation. For new technology fears, he'll sign up for a refresher course if necessary. For family pressure, he'll communicate updates regularly, so they understand he's making progress.

He also tries **Worksheet #5: "Early Warning System" (Maintaining Momentum and Relapse Prevention).** Gianni notes subtle signs of avoidance: sleeping in, scrolling aimlessly online, ignoring emails about job fairs. Once he detects these signals, he aims to set a small daily target, like sending one networking message or reading about an industry trend. This micro-step approach reduces the overwhelm.

Sustaining Accountability and Reinforcing Commitment

Gianni picks an old coworker, Franco, as an accountability buddy. Together they fill out **Worksheet #6: "Accountability Structure" (Strengthening Commitment).** Franco, also job hunting after layoffs, agrees to weekly video calls. They'll discuss steps taken, leads found, and obstacles faced. This mutual support can keep them from sinking into isolation.

He then sets up a **Maintenance Checklist** (Maintaining Momentum), listing daily or weekly tasks:

- Did he spend at least 30 minutes on skill-building or job research?

- Did he apply to at least one new position or make a networking contact per week?

- Did he update his progress log or check in with Franco?

This structured approach ensures small, consistent actions rather than waiting for bursts of motivation.

Addressing Setbacks and Self-Compassion

A couple of weeks in, Gianni applies for a mechanical design role. After an encouraging phone interview, he's turned down. Feeling crushed, he backslides for a few days, ignoring further job postings. The therapist suggests **Worksheet #8: "Turning Setbacks into Lessons" (Strengthening Commitment).** Gianni realises:

- **Trigger**: High hopes pinned on one interview.

- **Lesson**: Diversify applications and seek feedback from recruiters or the interviewer if possible.

- **Forward Step**: He'll keep exploring multiple leads, accept that rejections happen, and refine his pitch.

They also use **Worksheet #10: "Self-Compassion During Slips" (Maintaining Momentum).** Gianni writes a gentle statement: "This one 'no' doesn't define my entire career potential. I'm learning from each attempt." By framing it kindly, he avoids giving up altogether.

Monitoring Progress and Remaining Flexible

After a month, Gianni has discovered that local bike shops pay less than he hoped. Meanwhile, a manufacturing plant in a neighbouring town is hiring, but the role seems repetitive. He tries **Worksheet #9: "Flexible Goal Updates" (Maintaining Momentum).** Maybe he'll consider an alternative: short-term acceptance of a stable manufacturing job while pursuing part-time training for advanced mechanical design. That path maintains income while prepping for a more stimulating role later. Recognising he has an option helps quell panic.

He also references **Worksheet #4: "Reviewing Successes" (Maintaining Momentum)**:

- He's updated his résumé thoroughly.

- He's submitted four applications, got one interview, and extended his network by contacting three old colleagues.

- He's less anxious day to day because he has a routine.

Seeing these small wins reaffirms that he's not stagnant.

Preventing Complacency and Maintaining Long-Term Vision

Gianni's therapist prompts him to watch for complacency. If he lands a so-so job, he might forget his bigger dream. He checks **Worksheet #5: "Detecting Complacency" (Maintaining Momentum)**, noting:

- If he abandons skill-building or night courses, it might mean he's settling.

- If he stops networking, he might miss out on better opportunities.

Finally, they do a **Final Reflection** using **Worksheet #3: "Final Reflection" (Maintaining Momentum).** Gianni realises:

- **Before**: He was paralysed by fear post-layoff, lacking direction.

- **Now**: He's actively researching, applying, and learning new angles.

- **Main Takeaway**: A structured approach of small steps and consistent accountability counters hopelessness.

- **Future**: If he lands a transitional job, he'll keep training for a more satisfying position.

He leaves therapy feeling more capable, with a practical plan and an ongoing method to handle rejections or family worries. By systematically deploying MI worksheets across categories—engagement, focusing, evoking, commitment, and momentum—Gianni transforms a post-layoff crisis into a moment of exploration. His confidence grows as he realises these tools let him adapt, refine, and keep aiming for a job that aligns with his mechanical passions and financial needs.

Foundational Exercises

The Big Picture

The worksheets in this section target the **core principles** of MI. They are designed to help both novice and experienced therapists develop comfort with MI language and style, providing concrete strategies to reinforce essential skills. While each exercise can be adapted to various client situations, they are especially useful for establishing an initial framework for **empathetic, autonomy-supporting conversations**.

Worksheet 1: Active Listening Basics

Title
Active Listening Basics

Purpose
You learn to focus on your client's key messages, including feelings and aims. This exercise helps you pick out unspoken thoughts, making your client feel seen and heard.

The Rationale
Research by Rogers (1957) highlights the power of empathic listening in building trust. Tuning in to another person's core ideas and emotions can spark stronger engagement and willingness to share.

Step-by-Step Instructions

1. Ask your client to share a recent experience.
2. Maintain steady eye contact and calm posture.
3. Paraphrase what they say and notice any shifts in tone.
4. Validate their feelings, pointing out the emotions you sense.

Tips for Debriefing

- Encourage the client to share feedback on your listening style.
- Ask what felt most helpful.
- Highlight how accurate reflections boost connection.

Troubleshooting Common Challenges

- If the client seems guarded, use fewer questions and more gentle nods.
- If you catch your mind wandering, refocus on their words and body language.
- If the client is vague, softly encourage examples to clarify points.

Reflection Questions

- How did your client react when you paraphrased their words?
- Did you feel any urge to interrupt?

Real-Life Application

Brian, 25, spoke about conflict at work. While Brian talked, his therapist leaned forward and nodded. The therapist restated, "You're upset because your boss didn't recognise your effort." Brian confirmed that was true, then shared more details. Feeling heard, he became calmer and more open to talking about solutions. Active listening helped Brian feel understood, which strengthened trust.

Worksheet 2: Empathy in Action

Title
Empathy in Action

Purpose
You build genuine warmth by showing you truly understand the client's perspective. Empathy encourages them to open up about deeper worries and hopes.

The Rationale
According to Miller and Rollnick (2013), empathy is a key principle in Motivational Interviewing. It fosters trust and helps clients feel comfortable exploring challenges.

Step-by-Step Instructions

1. List possible empathetic statements (e.g., "It sounds like you felt disappointed.").
2. Practice saying each statement with a tone that matches the client's mood.
3. Pair body language cues (like leaning in) with your statements.

Tips for Debriefing

- Ask your client how they felt hearing your empathetic remarks.
- Explore any mismatch between your words and nonverbal signals.

Troubleshooting Common Challenges

- Forced empathy can sound fake. Slow down and think about the client's emotions first.

- If your tone is flat, try a gentle, caring style.

Reflection Questions

- Did the client's posture change when you used empathetic statements?
- How did you feel after offering empathy?

Real-Life Application
Maria, 40, felt stress about managing family duties. Her therapist said, "It seems you're worried about doing everything right." Maria relaxed and admitted she often felt overwhelmed. The therapist's kind tone and gentle nods convinced Maria she wasn't being judged. This motivated her to talk about possible coping steps.

Worksheet 3: Open-Ended Questioning Practice

Title
Open-Ended Questioning Practice

Purpose
You learn to invite clients to share their thoughts in detail. Open-ended prompts often uncover deeper insights and let the client guide the conversation.

The Rationale
Research by Miller and Rollnick (2013) shows that open-ended questions encourage clients to talk about their feelings and motivations, enhancing collaboration.

Step-by-Step Instructions

1. Create three open-ended questions for a scenario (e.g., "What led you to feel this way?").
2. Ask each question in a gentle tone.
3. Note which question sparked the longest or most personal response.
4. Reflect on how these questions differ from yes/no prompts.

Tips for Debriefing

- Discuss which question felt most natural to you and why.
- Explore how the client responded emotionally.

Troubleshooting Common Challenges

- If you slip into closed questions, pause and rephrase.
- If the client gives one-word answers, gently encourage them to expand.

Reflection Questions

- Which question revealed the strongest emotions?
- Did you notice any shift in the client's willingness to share?

Real-Life Application
Ravi, 28, came with performance stress. The therapist asked, "What do you think causes your nerves before a big presentation?" This question allowed Ravi to explain feelings of self-doubt. By avoiding yes/no language, the therapist uncovered more details about his anxious thoughts, paving the way for practical coping strategies.

Worksheet 4: Developing a Guiding Style

Title
Developing a Guiding Style

Purpose
You gain skill in steering the conversation without pushing advice. This style helps clients discover their own reasons to take action.

The Rationale
Miller and Rollnick (2013) highlight that guiding is different from directing or following. It promotes shared understanding and respects autonomy.

Step-by-Step Instructions

1. List two or three conversation starters that encourage insight (e.g., "How do you see this unfolding?").

2. Practise letting the client generate answers instead of immediately giving tips.
3. Note your feelings when you resist the urge to "fix" problems.
4. Summarise the client's thoughts to confirm you understand.

Tips for Debriefing

- Let the client reflect on the session's flow.
- Ask if they felt supported rather than led.

Troubleshooting Common Challenges

- If you slip into lecturing, pause and say, "Let me hear your thoughts first."
- If the client hesitates, offer gentle prompts like "What would you like to explore next?"

Reflection Questions

- Did you find it hard to hold back from giving direct advice?
- How did the client respond to your questions?

Real-Life Application

Lena, 35, wanted to handle family disagreements better. Her counsellor said, "Where do you think the main issue starts?" Lena realised she often felt guilt after arguments. By guiding rather than dictating, the counsellor let Lena form her own insights about patterns at home.

Worksheet 5: Reflective Listening for Emotions

Title
Reflective Listening for Emotions

Purpose
You improve your ability to detect underlying emotions in a client's story and echo them back, helping the client feel safe.

The Rationale

Rogers (1957) found that reflecting emotions deepens rapport, as it validates the client's experiences.

Step-by-Step Instructions

1. Invite the client to talk about a recent event.
2. Look for an emotion word ("sad," "worried").
3. Offer a reflection: "It sounds like that made you feel concerned."
4. Wait for the client to confirm or correct your guess.

Tips for Debriefing

- Ask how the client felt when you named the emotion.
- Reinforce that they can correct you if you misunderstand.

Troubleshooting Common Challenges

- If the client hesitates, try a softer reflection.
- If you repeatedly get the emotion wrong, apologise and ask for clarification.

Reflection Questions

- Did you sense the client relaxing after you reflected their feelings?
- How did naming the emotion affect the discussion?

Real-Life Application

Tariq, 42, described a tense office argument. He seemed frustrated but never used that word. The therapist reflected, "It sounds like you felt let down by your colleague." Tariq paused, nodded, and clarified he felt ignored. This opened the door to a deeper talk about unmet needs at work.

Worksheet 6: Exploring Autonomy

Title

Exploring Autonomy

Purpose
You help clients recognise their freedom to decide. This approach boosts ownership of change.

The Rationale
Self-determination research (Deci & Ryan, 2008) shows that clients who see choices as their own are more likely to follow through on goals.

Step-by-Step Instructions

1. Explain that the client holds the steering wheel in decisions.
2. Ask them to list reasons they appreciate having a choice.
3. Encourage them to think about who or what might affect these choices.
4. Discuss which choices feel most urgent or important.

Tips for Debriefing

- Remind the client that no one can force them to change.
- Ask how it feels to have full ownership of decisions.

Troubleshooting Common Challenges

- If the client is used to being told what to do, proceed slowly.
- If they doubt their own power, gently point out past examples where they made independent decisions.

Reflection Questions

- Did anything surprise you about acknowledging your autonomy?
- Which factors make choices feel easy or hard?

Real-Life Application
Joan, 50, felt stuck with her diet plan because her doctor insisted on strict rules. Through autonomy-focused discussion, Joan saw that she could choose how to adapt healthy eating in her daily life, boosting her sense of control and increasing her willingness to try changes.

Worksheet 7: Stages of Change Overview

Title
Stages of Change Overview

Purpose
You help clients pinpoint their current phase—whether they're just thinking or already taking steps—so they can plan next moves effectively.

The Rationale
Prochaska and DiClemente (1983) introduced the Stages of Change model. Identifying a client's stage shapes the best intervention approach.

Step-by-Step Instructions

1. Explain the stages: Precontemplation, Contemplation, Preparation, Action, Maintenance.
2. Ask the client to choose which stage fits them best now.
3. Discuss what might help them advance to the next level.
4. Brainstorm actions to fit their stage (e.g., gather information if still thinking).

Tips for Debriefing

- Encourage reflection on any past times they went through similar stages.
- Emphasise that it's normal to slip between stages.

Troubleshooting Common Challenges

- If the client feels stuck in a stage, brainstorm small, manageable steps.
- If they change stages quickly, revisit the model regularly.

Reflection Questions

- How does knowing your stage influence your confidence?
- Which stage felt surprising to you?

Real-Life Application
Aiden, 23, wasn't sure if he wanted to quit smoking. He identified as being in

Contemplation. By naming that stage, he realised he was still gathering info and wasn't ready to act. That helped him choose smaller steps, like researching options, rather than jumping straight to quitting.

Worksheet 8: Value Clarification

Title
Value Clarification

Purpose
You guide clients to list core personal principles and see how actions either match or conflict with these guiding ideas.

The Rationale
Sheldon and Kasser (1998) suggest that understanding personal values can create a stronger motivation to change when behaviour doesn't align with what matters most.

Step-by-Step Instructions

1. Ask the client to write five values (e.g., family, health, kindness).
2. Discuss how current habits support or go against these values.
3. Choose one or two values as top priority for the near future.
4. Brainstorm ways to bring behaviour closer to these highlighted values.

Tips for Debriefing

- Explore how it feels to see values in writing.
- Encourage the client to share which values carry the most emotional weight.

Troubleshooting Common Challenges

- If the client struggles to name values, prompt them to think about what they respect in others.
- If they list too many, help them focus on just a few.

Reflection Questions

- Which value did you find easiest to name?
- What first step can you try to live this value more fully?

Real-Life Application

Jen, 32, named honesty, health, and friendship as top values. She realised she ignored her health by skipping check-ups. By acknowledging this conflict, Jen felt inspired to schedule a doctor's visit and include more nutritious meals, drawing her actions closer to her stated value.

Worksheet 9: Change Ruler Introduction

Title

Change Ruler Introduction

Purpose

You assess how important, confident, and ready your client feels on a scale of 1–10. This quick measure shows where to focus your support.

The Rationale

Miller and Rollnick (2013) advocate the change ruler to clarify the client's readiness. It gives a tangible way to talk about motivation.

Step-by-Step Instructions

1. Draw three separate rulers, each numbered 1–10.
2. Label them: Importance, Confidence, and Readiness.
3. Ask the client to mark their current rating on each.
4. Explore what raised or lowered the rating.

Tips for Debriefing

- Prompt the client to reflect on times the number has been higher.
- Ask what small tweaks might boost the score by one point.

Troubleshooting Common Challenges

- If the client finds rating hard, suggest a simpler 1–5 scale.
- If the rating is 1, focus on exploring reasons for any interest at all.

Reflection Questions

- What factors keep your rating where it is?
- Which rating do you feel is easiest to improve?

Real-Life Application

Paul, 39, rated importance of quitting caffeine at 7, confidence at 4, and readiness at 5. Realising his confidence was lower, he decided to try smaller steps first, like replacing one cup of coffee with herbal tea. Over time, his confidence increased to 6.

Worksheet 10: Strength-Focused Exploration

Title

Strength-Focused Exploration

Purpose

You help clients remember times they have succeeded before. These successes can provide clues for handling new issues.

The Rationale

Bandura (1997) explains that recalling past triumphs boosts self-belief. This positivity can serve as a strong foundation for fresh goals.

Step-by-Step Instructions

1. Invite the client to list three moments they felt proud or achieved something meaningful.
2. Ask, "What skills did you use then?"
3. Brainstorm how those skills might apply to a current challenge.
4. Create a small plan to tap those strengths again.

Tips for Debriefing

- Reinforce how past wins show genuine ability.
- Ask the client to identify any similarities between old and new obstacles.

Troubleshooting Common Challenges

- If the client struggles to see strengths, gently probe for smaller wins.
- If they downplay achievements, reassure them that every success matters.

Reflection Questions

- What new challenge could benefit from your listed strengths?
- Which past win still brings a sense of pride?

Real-Life Application
Kevin, 27, recalled how he learned to swim despite a fear of water. He used patience, seeking advice from a friend, and steady practice. Now facing anxiety about job interviews, he realised the same skills—asking for help and practising—could ease his interview nerves.

Worksheet 11: Summarising the Session

Title
Summarising the Session

Purpose
You make sure the client feels heard, and you capture the key points before wrapping up. Clear summaries boost clarity and shared understanding.

The Rationale
Miller and Rollnick (2013) note that regular summaries help maintain focus, showing the client you value their words.

Step-by-Step Instructions

1. Listen for main themes during the conversation.
2. Near the session's end, say, "Let me briefly outline what we covered."

3. Include the client's goals, emotions, and any next steps.
4. Ask for feedback or corrections.

Tips for Debriefing

- Encourage the client to fill in missed details or correct anything.
- Note how summarising might clarify confusion.

Troubleshooting Common Challenges

- If you forget key details, ask the client to repeat important points.
- If time is short, offer a quick bullet-list summary.

Reflection Questions

- Did the summary help the client feel validated?
- Did you notice any new insights while summarising?

Real-Life Application
Kim, 26, talked about career uncertainty. The therapist summarised: "You feel stuck in a job that isn't fulfilling, and you want to explore new training options." Kim nodded and mentioned she also felt worried about finances, prompting the therapist to adjust the summary to include financial anxieties.

Worksheet 12: Affirmation Enhancement

Title
Affirmation Enhancement

Purpose
You learn how to highlight a client's unique qualities in meaningful ways. Specific affirmations can spark optimism and self-belief.

The Rationale
Research by Seligman (2011) suggests that authentic praise helps people recognise

their potential, fuelling growth. Affirmations show clients that you see their progress and strengths.

Step-by-Step Instructions

1. Write three specific statements describing the client's positive traits (e.g., "You showed bravery.").
2. Double-check each statement focuses on a behaviour or quality, not a shallow compliment.
3. Deliver them calmly, noticing the client's reaction.
4. Invite the client to say how they feel hearing these affirmations.

Tips for Debriefing

- Let the client share if any statement felt more impactful.
- If they seem uncomfortable, confirm that it's okay to accept praise.

Troubleshooting Common Challenges

- Avoid generic phrases ("You're great!").
- If the client downplays the affirmation, ask gentle questions about past accomplishments.

Reflection Questions

- Which affirmation resonated with you the most?
- Did these statements shift your outlook?

Real-Life Application

Rina, 41, struggled with self-doubt. Her therapist affirmed her steady dedication to her family, saying, "You consistently show up for your children's school events, which reveals loyalty and love." Rina teared up, realising she was stronger than she thought.

Worksheet 13: Listening with Curiosity

Title
Listening with Curiosity

Purpose
You grow more open-minded by swapping quick fixes for thoughtful questions. This invites the client to explore deeper layers of their story.

The Rationale
Barrett-Lennard (1993) says that genuine curiosity fosters a non-judgmental space. Clients who sense open curiosity feel safer discussing painful topics.

Step-by-Step Instructions

1. Identify a moment when you usually give direct advice.
2. Instead, form an open question about the client's viewpoint.
3. Practise active listening, avoiding mental planning for "the answer."
4. Summarise what you heard, highlighting any new insights.

Tips for Debriefing

- Share whether you felt tension holding back from giving solutions.
- Note if your interest encouraged the client to go deeper.

Troubleshooting Common Challenges

- If you catch yourself jumping in with a solution, pause and reframe into a question.
- If the client demands answers, remind them you want to hear their thoughts first.

Reflection Questions

- Did your approach uncover any details you might have missed otherwise?
- How did the client respond to your curious stance?

Real-Life Application
Kay, 29, asked her therapist how to fix her relationship quickly. Instead of providing a list of steps, the therapist asked, "What do you think triggered this recent conflict?" Kay realised she had deeper resentments to work through. This shift led her to consider new insights rather than seeking a single remedy.

Worksheet 14: Exploring Pros and Cons

Title
Exploring Pros and Cons

Purpose
You help clients see benefits and downsides of changing or staying the same. This often clarifies mixed feelings.

The Rationale
Janis and Mann (1977) suggest that weighing advantages and drawbacks can reduce indecision. It encourages a more balanced view of the situation.

Step-by-Step Instructions

1. Split a page into two columns for pros and cons of making a change.
2. Add a second set of columns for pros and cons of NOT making that change.
3. Ask the client to reflect on each item's importance.
4. Discuss any patterns that emerge.

Tips for Debriefing

- Point out if certain pros or cons carry strong emotional weight.
- Encourage the client to prioritise each item to find key factors.

Troubleshooting Common Challenges

- If the list feels too big, highlight the top few on each side.
- If the client is stuck, prompt them to consider past outcomes.

Reflection Questions

- Were you surprised by any pros or cons?
- Which factor is the biggest influencer on your next step?

Real-Life Application

Jon, 34, debated leaving his job. He saw that staying offered stability but brought boredom. Changing might bring adventure yet risked failure. After listing his pros and cons, Jon realised the boredom was affecting his mood more than he first thought, making him more open to exploring other work.

Worksheet 15: Cultural Sensitivity Check

Title

Cultural Sensitivity Check

Purpose

You ensure you honour a client's cultural or family background. Awareness of these elements can shape more respectful communication.

The Rationale

Sue & Sue (2012) emphasise that cultural contexts influence how people see themselves and respond to therapy. Sensitivity encourages trust.

Step-by-Step Instructions

1. Ask the client to share important traditions or values.
2. Listen for how these might affect their decision-making.
3. Adjust your language and pace to respect their style.
4. Invite the client to correct you if you misunderstand any aspect of their culture.

Tips for Debriefing

- Check if the client feels comfortable discussing culture in sessions.
- Affirm that you appreciate learning from them.

Troubleshooting Common Challenges

- If you worry about unintentionally offending, ask the client to guide you.
- If the client hesitates, remind them this is a safe space.

Reflection Questions

- Did cultural factors change how the client framed their concerns?
- How did you adapt your approach?

Real-Life Application
A therapist worked with Rosa, 45, who values extended family involvement. The therapist invited her to explain how family gatherings shape her stress. By respecting her background, the therapist and Rosa found ways to include family support rather than viewing it as a barrier.

Worksheet 16: Mindful Presence

Title
Mindful Presence

Purpose
You centre yourself before a session, avoiding distractions. This lets you offer clients your full attention.

The Rationale
Kabat-Zinn (1990) suggests that mindfulness techniques reduce mental chatter, improving the ability to remain steady and attentive.

Step-by-Step Instructions

1. Sit quietly for one minute before meeting the client.
2. Focus on slow, steady breathing.
3. Notice your thoughts without clinging to them, then bring attention back to your breath.
4. Enter the session feeling calmer and more grounded.

Tips for Debriefing

- Reflect with a colleague on any shift you felt in your concentration.
- Encourage the client to notice your calm energy.

Troubleshooting Common Challenges

- If the space is busy, find a quiet corner or use noise-cancelling earphones.
- If your mind races, it's okay—gently return to focusing on breathing.

Reflection Questions

- Did you observe any improvement in how you listened during the session?
- How might a brief pause benefit your overall day?

Real-Life Application
Pat, a busy therapist, tried a one-minute pause before a high-stress appointment. After gently focusing on breathing, he noticed less restlessness when the client arrived. He asked more thoughtful questions and felt more balanced throughout the session.

Worksheet 17: Resisting the Righting Reflex

Title
Resisting the Righting Reflex

Purpose
You learn to avoid trying to "fix" the client right away, instead staying collaborative and curious.

The Rationale
Miller and Rollnick (2013) note that well-meaning helpers often jump to solve problems. Holding back fosters a client's self-motivation.

Step-by-Step Instructions

1. Write down situations where you felt the urge to give direct advice.

2. Reframe each urge as an open question or empathic statement.
3. Practise using these new phrases in role-play or real sessions.
4. Track how clients respond differently.

Tips for Debriefing

- Check with a colleague if you find it hard not to fix issues.
- Celebrate small steps in letting clients guide themselves.

Troubleshooting Common Challenges

- If a client explicitly asks for direct answers, you can still first ask about their ideas.
- If you revert to fixing, gently note it and try again.

Reflection Questions

- How did it feel to hold back from providing solutions?
- Did the client appear more empowered?

Real-Life Application
Cara, a social worker, usually offered step-by-step solutions. After this worksheet, she paused instead and asked, "What do you think could help most right now?" Her clients seemed more invested in brainstorming their own ideas.

Worksheet 18: Change Talk Bingo

Title
Change Talk Bingo

Purpose
You become more aware of words or phrases that suggest a client is ready for change, like "I wish," "I need," or "I could."

The Rationale

Miller and Rollnick (2013) define "change talk" as statements expressing desire, ability, reasons, or need for change. Spotting them guides your response.

Step-by-Step Instructions

1. Create a bingo card with typical change talk phrases in each square.
2. During the session, gently mark the phrases you hear.
3. Reflect each phrase back to the client to encourage more discussion.
4. Tally the phrases at the end.

Tips for Debriefing

- Show enthusiasm whenever you hear a change talk phrase.
- Let the client know these words signal possible motivation.

Troubleshooting Common Challenges

- If you rarely hear any phrases, ask open questions to spark them.
- If the client uses them but doesn't expand, reflect or paraphrase to dig deeper.

Reflection Questions

- Which phrases popped up the most?
- Did highlighting these words inspire the client to keep talking?

Real-Life Application

Greg, a counsellor, used a "bingo" list. His client said, "I really want to have more energy" and "I might try cutting back on fast food." Greg noted two squares and repeated them back: "You want more energy, and you might reduce fast food." The client felt heard and explored changes further.

Worksheet 19: Body Language Awareness

Title

Body Language Awareness

Purpose

You learn how your posture, facial expressions, and gestures affect the session's atmosphere.

The Rationale

Mehrabian (1972) highlights how nonverbal signals carry a large portion of interpersonal messages.

Step-by-Step Instructions

1. Ask a colleague or friend to observe one session, focusing on your body language.
2. Have them note if you cross your arms, avoid eye contact, or lean away.
3. Check your notes afterward and pick one habit to adjust.
4. Practise a more open stance in future sessions.

Tips for Debriefing

- Ask the client how they felt about your nonverbal cues.
- Talk with a peer for feedback on any posture improvements.

Troubleshooting Common Challenges

- If you find it tough to maintain open body language, set small goals (like uncrossing arms).
- If you feel awkward at first, remember that practice helps it become natural.

Reflection Questions

- Did the shift in posture change the client's comfort level?
- How did you feel in your body when adjusting your stance?

Real-Life Application

Patrice, a therapist, often sat with arms crossed and seemed tense. A colleague's notes revealed this might appear defensive. Patrice focused on resting hands on her lap and tilting slightly forward. She noticed clients started talking more and seemed more at ease.

Worksheet 20: Self-Evaluation of MI Skills

Title
Self-Evaluation of MI Skills

Purpose
You reflect on your strengths and areas to grow within Motivational Interviewing. Honest self-review helps you enhance your techniques.

The Rationale
Miller and Rollnick (2013) encourage ongoing self-assessment to stay on track with MI principles like empathy, collaboration, and evoking change talk.

Step-by-Step Instructions

1. List key MI skills: open-ended questions, reflections, affirmations, summaries, evoking change talk.
2. Rate your proficiency on a scale of 1–5 for each.
3. Consider session feedback or peer observation to refine your rating.
4. Choose one skill to focus on improving.

Tips for Debriefing

- Share your self-ratings with a trusted colleague or supervisor if possible.
- Encourage the client to give feedback on how supported they feel.

Troubleshooting Common Challenges

- If you feel discouraged by low ratings, treat it as a chance to grow.
- If you overrate your skills, keep an open mind for feedback from others.

Reflection Questions

- Which skill did you score highest? Why do you think that is?
- Which skill do you plan to improve next?

Real-Life Application
Megan, a counsellor, scored herself low on eliciting change talk. She set a personal

target: "This week, I'll reflect any sign of change talk rather than skip past it." After one week, Megan saw better client engagement and felt more confident in her MI approach.

Worksheet 21: Double-Sided Reflections

Title
Double-Sided Reflections

Purpose
You practise capturing both sides of a client's ambivalence in one statement, showing empathy for their mixed feelings.

The Rationale
Miller and Rollnick (2013) describe double-sided reflections as a skill that validates conflicting emotions, guiding clients to feel understood rather than judged.

Step-by-Step Instructions

1. Listen for at least two contrasting feelings the client has about a topic.
2. Form a reflection that includes both sides: "On one hand… yet on the other…"
3. Deliver it calmly, checking for accuracy.
4. Note the client's response and see if they clarify or resolve some tension.

Tips for Debriefing

- Encourage the client to confirm or correct each side of the reflection.
- Reinforce that conflicted feelings are normal.

Troubleshooting Common Challenges

- If the client feels invalidated, recheck your reflection.
- If they're highly emotional, consider simpler reflections first.

Reflection Questions

- Did the client feel relief at having their ambivalence acknowledged?
- Did your reflection lead to a clearer understanding?

Real-Life Application
Esther, 29, wanted to relocate for work but also feared leaving friends behind. Her therapist said, "You crave new career opportunities, yet you worry about losing important relationships." Esther relaxed, realising it was okay to hold two opposing views.

Worksheet 22: Confidence Boosting Prompts

Title
Confidence Boosting Prompts

Purpose
You use simple statements that encourage clients to believe in their capabilities. This helps them see their potential to handle the next step.

The Rationale
Bandura (1997) links confidence (self-efficacy) with better outcomes. Small prompts can nudge people to try challenging tasks.

Step-by-Step Instructions

1. Brainstorm three quick phrases that remind clients of their strengths (e.g., "You've tackled tough tasks before.").
2. Write them down and keep them visible.
3. In sessions, weave these prompts into conversation when you see hesitancy.
4. Ask clients how it feels to hear these reminders.

Tips for Debriefing

- Encourage the client to adopt some prompts as self-talk.
- Validate any skepticism, yet gently reinforce their past successes.

Troubleshooting Common Challenges

- If prompts feel forced, adjust the wording to suit the client's personality.
- If the client rejects them, explore underlying doubts.

Reflection Questions

- Which prompt seemed to resonate the most?
- Did they mention any shifts in mood or determination?

Real-Life Application
Dean, 50, felt stuck in therapy, doubting he could improve. His counsellor often said, "You've solved big problems before." Over time, Dean began repeating this phrase to himself at home, and he noticed a jump in his willingness to try new coping methods.

Worksheet 23: Using Silence Wisely

Title
Using Silence Wisely

Purpose
You practise allowing pauses during sessions, giving the client space to reflect and speak at their own pace.

The Rationale
Hill (2010) notes that quiet moments can invite deeper conversation and let the client process feelings more fully.

Step-by-Step Instructions

1. When the client finishes a thought, wait a few seconds before responding.
2. Observe if they continue or add more details.
3. If they remain quiet, gently ask, "Is there more on your mind?"
4. Reflect on how the pause changed the session's flow.

Tips for Debriefing

- Check if the client felt awkward or at ease with the silence.

- Discuss how this space opened new insights or feelings.

Troubleshooting Common Challenges

- If you get anxious, focus on your breath to stay calm.
- If the client seems uneasy, assure them they can speak whenever ready.

Reflection Questions

- Did the pause lead to richer sharing?
- How did you manage your own discomfort?

Real-Life Application
Talia, a therapist, noticed her frequent talking sometimes interrupted clients. She started a practice of counting to five after each client statement. One client used that pause to add a key detail about their childhood trauma. This opened a more meaningful dialogue.

Worksheet 24: Identify Client Triggers

Title
Identify Client Triggers

Purpose
You help the client detect events or feelings that spark harmful behaviours or distress. Recognising triggers is a step toward prevention.

The Rationale
Stimulus-response models (Skinner, 1953) suggest that awareness of cues can break negative cycles. Identifying triggers makes it easier to plan new responses.

Step-by-Step Instructions

1. Ask the client to list situations, people, or emotions that tend to set off the problematic behaviour.
2. Sort them into "high risk" vs. "low risk."

3. Brainstorm safer ways to handle or avoid these triggers.
4. Select one or two high-risk triggers to work on first.

Tips for Debriefing

- Validate the client's feelings if triggers involve sensitive topics.
- Encourage them to share personal insights on how triggers develop.

Troubleshooting Common Challenges

- If the client can't identify triggers, suggest they keep a daily log.
- If triggers are too numerous, focus on the top few that cause the most trouble.

Reflection Questions

- Which trigger did you find easiest to name?
- How might planning ahead help you manage these triggers?

Real-Life Application
Jake, 38, noticed that late-night boredom triggered overeating. By naming that as a high-risk period, he decided to schedule engaging tasks during evenings. This simple change reduced his snack binges and lifted his mood.

Worksheet 25: Foundations of Collaboration

Title
Foundations of Collaboration

Purpose
You create an equal partnership with your client, ensuring they have input in every part of the counselling process.

The Rationale
Carl Rogers (1957) emphasises that shared respect fosters trust. Clients who collaborate feel more motivated to participate fully.

Step-by-Step Instructions

1. Start each session by asking, "What would you like to focus on today?"
2. When you propose activities, ask for the client's feedback or modifications.
3. Encourage the client to shape homework tasks.
4. Check in frequently, "How does this approach feel to you?"

Tips for Debriefing

- Ask the client to rate their sense of involvement.
- Reinforce that their voice is central in setting goals and methods.

Troubleshooting Common Challenges

- If the client defers too much, remind them that their input is valuable.
- If they seem overwhelmed, offer a brief menu of possible options.

Reflection Questions

- Did the client engage more when they co-created the plan?
- Which part of collaboration felt new or unusual to you?

Real-Life Application

Mia, 46, often expected the therapist to lead. By asking Mia to pick topics and shape her own homework, she began taking ownership of her progress. She felt proud when she completed tasks she had helped design.

Worksheet 26: Shifting from Expert to Ally

Title
Shifting from Expert to Ally

Purpose
You notice moments when you slip into the "expert" role and learn how to return to a more supportive, equal dynamic.

The Rationale

Miller and Rollnick (2013) highlight that clients often respond better when you act as a guide rather than an authority.

Step-by-Step Instructions

1. Recall a recent session where you gave plenty of advice.
2. Ask yourself, "How could I have encouraged the client to share more ideas?"
3. Write alternate phrases (e.g., "What do you think about…?").
4. Practise these new lines in your next session.

Tips for Debriefing

- Compare how the session feels when you position yourself as a collaborator.
- Reflect on moments you unknowingly become the "teacher."

Troubleshooting Common Challenges

- If you worry about not being helpful, focus on listening more.
- If the client expects you to be the authority, gently clarify that their insights matter the most.

Reflection Questions

- Did you see any difference in the client's engagement?
- How did you feel offering less direct instruction?

Real-Life Application

Omar, a seasoned therapist, realised he often lectured clients on coping strategies. During a session with Mark, he deliberately asked, "How do you think you might handle this anxiety?" Mark offered his own ideas, leading to a shared plan that felt more personal.

Worksheet 27: Mirroring Key Words

Title
Mirroring Key Words

Purpose
You underline the words with emotional weight so the client realises those points matter. This fosters deeper dialogue.

The Rationale
Miller and Rollnick (2013) show that clients respond well when therapists reflect their own phrases, feeling validated and encouraged to expand.

Step-by-Step Instructions

1. Listen for words that hold strong feeling (e.g., "shame," "trapped," "hopeful").
2. Repeat those words in your reflection: "You felt 'trapped' in that situation."
3. Pause and see if the client adds more details.
4. Integrate these words in later summaries.

Tips for Debriefing

- Note how the client's mood shifts when hearing their own words back.
- Confirm you haven't misheard or twisted the meaning.

Troubleshooting Common Challenges

- If you repeat a word incorrectly, let the client correct you.
- If it feels awkward, start small by mirroring one word per session.

Reflection Questions

- Did the client elaborate more when you used their key terms?
- Which words carried the strongest emotions?

Real-Life Application
Lucy, 29, said she felt "ignored" at home. Her counsellor repeated, "Ignored?" Lucy took a deep breath and went on to explain how she often felt invisible in her family. This reflection helped Lucy open up about her childhood experiences.

Worksheet 28: Understanding Resistance

Title
Understanding Resistance

Purpose
You explore possible reasons clients might push back or seem reluctant. Recognising the causes can help you respond calmly.

The Rationale
Rollnick, Miller, and Butler (2008) suggest that resistance is a signal to adjust your approach, not confront harder.

Step-by-Step Instructions

1. Write down different forms of resistance (e.g., denial, argument).
2. Note common triggers that prompt resistance (e.g., feeling rushed).
3. Plan empathetic statements: "It sounds like this is tough for you right now."
4. Practise responding with curiosity rather than debate.

Tips for Debriefing

- Reflect on whether your style might be adding pressure.
- Ask the client what would make them more comfortable.

Troubleshooting Common Challenges

- If tension grows, slow down and shift to empathic listening.
- If the client refuses to engage, respect their readiness and propose smaller steps.

Reflection Questions

- Which type of resistance do you encounter most often?
- How can you change your style to address it?

Real-Life Application
A therapist noticed that when discussing finances, Henry, 45, shut down. Rather than pushing, the therapist said, "It seems really upsetting to talk about money. I wonder if

we need to slow down and do this at a pace that feels safer to you." Henry eventually admitted he felt judged in past experiences, and they worked on a gentler plan.

Worksheet 29: Allowing Space for Emotions

Title
Allowing Space for Emotions

Purpose
You encourage clients to experience and name intense feelings without rushing to soothe them or shut them down.

The Rationale
Greenberg (2002) notes that validating emotions lets clients process them fully, which can lead to deeper self-understanding.

Step-by-Step Instructions

1. After the client names a strong feeling, invite them to sit with it for a moment.
2. Ask gentle follow-ups like "Where do you feel that in your body?"
3. Reflect back any words or images they use.
4. Assure them that strong feelings are acceptable and can reveal valuable insights.

Tips for Debriefing

- Normalise tears or anger, mentioning it's okay to express them here.
- Check if the client wants a short grounding technique afterward.

Troubleshooting Common Challenges

- If the client panics, offer gentle reassurance and slow breathing.
- If they shut down, respect their pace and avoid forcing deeper exploration.

Reflection Questions

- Did naming the emotion help it feel more manageable?
- How did you feel holding space for strong emotions?

Real-Life Application

Darius, 26, felt deep sadness about a recent breakup. His therapist gently asked where he felt it in his body. Darius placed a hand on his chest and wept. By not rushing him, the therapist allowed that wave of emotion to pass, and Darius later said he felt lighter and clearer.

Worksheet 30: Question Tree

Title
Question Tree

Purpose
You build a branching flow of possible follow-up questions, improving your ability to respond dynamically to clients' statements.

The Rationale
Effective questioning, as described by Egan (2013), can reveal root concerns. A structured approach ensures you stay flexible yet focused.

Step-by-Step Instructions

1. Draw a tree with a trunk: the client's main statement.
2. Branch off with possible open-ended questions.
3. Keep branching out as each question may lead to deeper follow-up.
4. Practise with a sample scenario.

Tips for Debriefing

- Reflect on which branch gave you the richest information.
- Ask if the client found the exploration helpful or overwhelming.

Troubleshooting Common Challenges

- If you get stuck on one branch, ask a different open-ended question.
- If it becomes too complicated, pick one branch and follow it gently.

Reflection Questions

- Did you discover any surprising path on your question tree?
- How did the client react to your deeper inquiries?

Real-Life Application
Sara, a trainee therapist, created a question tree for a client worried about career paths. One branch focused on the client's frustration at work, leading to a memory of feeling unappreciated by a parent. This path uncovered an emotional thread that shaped current decisions.

Worksheet 31: Goal Visualization

Title
Goal Visualization

Purpose
You invite clients to imagine a future where they have handled their challenges successfully, boosting hope and direction.

The Rationale
Bandura (1997) notes that picturing success can strengthen self-belief, leading to more consistent effort.

Step-by-Step Instructions

1. Ask the client to close their eyes (if comfortable) and picture themselves after achieving a key goal.
2. Prompt details: "What do you see, hear, or feel in this future?"
3. Encourage them to describe the vision out loud or sketch it.
4. Connect these images to next steps in real life.

Tips for Debriefing

- Ask what surprised them about their own vision.
- Emphasise that small steps today can build toward that positive image.

Troubleshooting Common Challenges

- If the client has trouble visualising, let them describe it in words or use a written narrative.
- If it triggers anxiety, gently slow down and remind them it's just an exercise.

Reflection Questions

- Did this mental picture increase your motivation?
- How can you use this vision during tough moments?

Real-Life Application
Sam, 24, pictured himself feeling calm and proud after finishing his nursing degree. He described walking across the graduation stage, hearing cheers, and feeling confident. This vision reminded him why his studies mattered, and he became more committed to daily revision.

Worksheet 32: Recognising Small Wins

Title
Recognising Small Wins

Purpose
You help clients track little achievements, reinforcing the sense that gradual progress is still progress.

The Rationale
Locke and Latham (2002) found that celebrating small milestones creates momentum and boosts motivation for bigger goals.

Step-by-Step Instructions

1. Give the client a short log to record one achievement per day, no matter how small.
2. Review them at each session.
3. Ask, "How did you create this small success?"
4. Discuss how these little steps add up.

Tips for Debriefing

- Praise the consistency of logging wins, even if they seem minor.
- Notice patterns in when or how successes happen.

Troubleshooting Common Challenges

- If the client forgets to log, suggest setting reminders.
- If they minimise their wins, remind them each step counts.

Reflection Questions

- Did focusing on small victories shift your attitude?
- Which daily achievement felt most satisfying?

Real-Life Application

Felicia, 33, wrote down that she refused a second dessert one evening. Though it seemed tiny, she realised it was a positive step toward healthier habits. As she kept logging such decisions, Felicia felt encouraged to continue making better choices.

Worksheet 33: Learning from Lapses

Title
Learning from Lapses

Purpose
You explore a setback or slip in behaviour, transforming it from a defeat into a chance to learn and adjust.

The Rationale
Marlatt and Gordon (1985) suggest that slips are common in any change process. Understanding them fosters resilience.

Step-by-Step Instructions

1. Ask the client to recount the lapse without shame.
2. Identify what triggered it and how they felt right before.
3. Note any positive steps they took, even if small.
4. Brainstorm strategies to prevent or handle similar lapses in the future.

Tips for Debriefing

- Emphasise that a lapse doesn't cancel all progress.
- Explore how the client can regain momentum quickly.

Troubleshooting Common Challenges

- If the client is overwhelmed by guilt, offer empathy and refocus on what they learned.
- If they treat the lapse as total failure, remind them that growth can involve ups and downs.

Reflection Questions

- What did this slip teach you about your triggers or coping skills?
- How might you respond differently next time?

Real-Life Application
Karen, 37, broke her promise to cut down on social media when stress hit. After reflection, she saw that feeling lonely spurred her to scroll aimlessly. She decided to keep a list of supportive friends to call when stress rises, aiming to avoid mindless scrolling.

Worksheet 34: Language of Partnership

Title
Language of Partnership

Purpose
You enhance the sense of working side by side with the client by using inclusive phrasing and encouraging them to co-create solutions.

The Rationale
Miller and Rollnick (2013) emphasize partnership language ("We can figure this out together") to inspire collaboration and respect.

Step-by-Step Instructions

1. Write a list of partnership phrases: "Let's consider...," "How do you feel about...," "What do you think of...?"
2. Practise weaving these phrases into your sessions.
3. Notice how the client's attitude changes when they hear inclusive language.
4. Encourage the client to respond with their own ideas.

Tips for Debriefing

- Discuss if the client felt more involved.
- Watch for a shift in their openness or positivity.

Troubleshooting Common Challenges

- If the client still wants you to lead entirely, gently remind them of their role.
- If you forget partnership language, keep a visible reminder.

Reflection Questions

- Did your wording help the client feel more at ease or in charge?
- Which phrase did you find easiest to use?

Real-Life Application
Cameron, a counsellor, replaced "Here's what you should do" with "How about we explore this idea?" Clients responded by offering more personal solutions, feeling they had a voice in creating their own plans.

Worksheet 35: Emotion-Focused Journaling

Title
Emotion-Focused Journaling

Purpose
You encourage clients to track their feelings daily, noting what sparks them and how they respond.

The Rationale
Pennebaker (1997) found that writing about emotions can lessen distress and boost mental health by promoting insight.

Step-by-Step Instructions

1. Hand out a simple daily journal template.
2. Ask clients to note each key feeling of the day and its trigger.
3. Include space for how they reacted and any coping skill they used.
4. Discuss patterns or surprises during the next session.

Tips for Debriefing

- Ask if writing helped them spot triggers faster.
- Validate any strong emotions that surfaced.

Troubleshooting Common Challenges

- If journaling feels tedious, encourage short bullet points.
- If they skip days, ask about practical ways to fit journaling into their routine.

Reflection Questions

- Did writing down your emotions help you see any trends?
- Which emotion showed up most often?

Real-Life Application

Ashley, 36, noticed she felt anxious each morning before checking emails. By keeping a journal, she discovered this anxiety came from a fear of negative feedback. Over time, she prepared herself with short breathing exercises before opening her inbox.

Worksheet 36: Inviting Autonomy

Title
Inviting Autonomy

Purpose
You highlight the client's right to make personal decisions, freeing them from external pressure and improving commitment to change.

The Rationale
Deci and Ryan (2008) show that when individuals sense genuine choice, they feel more motivated to act on it.

Step-by-Step Instructions

1. Use statements like, "It's up to you how you want to proceed."
2. Ask them to consider possible paths forward, even unusual options.
3. Respect any hesitations and ask if they want to revisit those ideas later.
4. Reinforce that they can revise choices at any time.

Tips for Debriefing

- See if the client feels empowered or overwhelmed.
- Offer gentle guidance if they struggle with unlimited choices.

Troubleshooting Common Challenges

- If the client is used to rigid guidance, this new approach may feel foreign.
- If they freeze at too many options, scale back to a few clear ones.

Reflection Questions

- Did realising you have a choice change your sense of control?
- Which path feels most appealing right now?

Real-Life Application
Brett, 48, often felt pressured by others to manage his health. Hearing "It's really your decision" from his therapist made Brett see that he could choose a method that suited him best, like starting a low-impact exercise routine instead of a gym membership he disliked.

Worksheet 37: Linking Strengths to Goals

Title
Linking Strengths to Goals

Purpose
You guide clients to connect personal assets—like creativity or discipline—to a specific short-term target, reinforcing their ability to succeed.

The Rationale
Bandura (1997) underscores that believing in your own skill set makes goals feel more realistic and less intimidating.

Step-by-Step Instructions

1. Ask the client to choose one short-term goal (e.g., cook healthier meals this week).
2. Identify one or two strengths (e.g., organisation, curiosity).
3. Brainstorm how these strengths can be used in achieving the chosen goal.
4. Encourage them to create a quick action plan.

Tips for Debriefing

- Remind them that success isn't about being perfect but leveraging their natural abilities.
- Celebrate even small progress as evidence of their strengths.

Troubleshooting Common Challenges

- If the client struggles to identify strengths, offer hints from previous sessions.
- If the goal is too broad, break it into smaller steps.

Reflection Questions

- How did your strengths help you with today's tasks?
- Did using these strengths boost your confidence?

Real-Life Application
Louise, 34, wanted to start jogging but hesitated. She realised she was good at planning, so she made a simple schedule for three short jogs per week. Putting that organising strength to use made it easier to follow through.

Worksheet 38: Motivation Pie Chart

Title
Motivation Pie Chart

Purpose
You map out different influences—like social support, personal desires, or financial needs—to see how they shape motivation.

The Rationale
Visualising motivation (Miller & Rollnick, 2013) helps clients grasp the relative power of each factor. This clarity guides better planning.

Step-by-Step Instructions

1. Draw a circle and divide it into slices that represent each source of motivation (friends, personal health, finances).
2. Label the size of each slice based on importance.
3. Discuss which slices could be grown or shrunk to foster lasting change.
4. Look for imbalances or missing elements.

Tips for Debriefing

- Ask if certain slices feel surprising in size.
- Explore how to balance or expand slices that matter most.

Troubleshooting Common Challenges

- If it's hard to divide by percentages, ask for approximate areas.
- If the client sees a tiny slice for personal desire, explore how to increase it.

Reflection Questions

- Which slice do you want to strengthen first?
- Which slice already seems to help you the most?

Real-Life Application
Nora, 29, discovered that pleasing her family took up half her chart, leaving little space for her own well-being. She decided to focus more on personal health by setting boundaries. Adjusting her "family approval" slice helped her see the need for self-care.

Worksheet 39: Shared Decision Roadmap

Title
Shared Decision Roadmap

Purpose
You co-create a plan for the session or the overall therapy journey, making sure the client feels a strong sense of ownership.

The Rationale
Miller and Rollnick (2013) advocate involving clients in planning to nurture engagement and accountability.

Step-by-Step Instructions

1. Ask, "What do you hope to accomplish today?"

2. Outline the key topics or goals together on a sheet.
3. Assign each step to you, the client, or both.
4. Review at the end of the session to see what was covered and what remains.

Tips for Debriefing

- Check if the client felt included in shaping the plan.
- Encourage them to suggest changes if something feels off.

Troubleshooting Common Challenges

- If the client is unsure, offer gentle suggestions but let them decide.
- If you run out of time, carry over leftover items to the next session.

Reflection Questions

- Did having a roadmap help keep the session on track?
- How did you feel about taking an active role in planning?

Real-Life Application
Luke, 31, often arrived at therapy unsure what to discuss. With a shared roadmap, he identified improving sleep and managing stress as top goals. They agreed to tackle sleep first and revisit stress later. This structure gave Luke clarity and direction.

Worksheet 40: Practitioner Reflective Practice

Title
Practitioner Reflective Practice

Purpose
You set aside time after each session to note what went well, what felt challenging, and how you can refine your style.

The Rationale
Schön (1983) emphasises reflective practice as a key to professional growth. It encourages adapting to client needs and improving methods.

Step-by-Step Instructions

1. Right after the session, jot down a quick summary of what happened.
2. Reflect on any moments you felt stuck or uneasy.
3. List one thing you did effectively and one area that needs fine-tuning.
4. Decide on one small goal for your next session.

Tips for Debriefing

- If you have a supervisor or peer, discuss your notes together.
- Keep track of patterns over time to see progress.

Troubleshooting Common Challenges

- If time is limited, stick to a simple template.
- If you feel discouraged, recall that all practitioners continue to grow their skills.

Reflection Questions

- What did you learn about your style today?
- Did anything surprise you about your client's reaction?

Real-Life Application
Marcie, a new counsellor, used a short reflection sheet after each appointment. She noticed she often spoke too quickly during heated moments. By writing it down and planning to slow her speech next time, she saw a steady improvement in her rapport with clients.

As you continue exploring these 40 worksheets, keep in mind that steady use and practice of these tools strengthens your MI approach. You will likely see your clients respond with more openness, self-awareness, and readiness to tackle the steps ahead.

Engaging and Building Rapport

This category focuses on creating a warm, safe environment where clients feel comfortable sharing. Worksheets here guide you in forming genuine connections, exploring the client's interests, and setting a supportive tone. A strong therapeutic bond paves the way for honest dialogue and deeper exploration.

Worksheet 1: First Impressions

The Purpose
You improve how you welcome clients by focusing on the setting and your own posture. This creates a calmer, inviting start.

The Rationale
Research by Hill (2010) shows that environment and initial body language shape how open clients feel in therapy. A well-prepared space reduces anxiety and builds safety.

Step-by-Step Instructions

1. Assess lighting, temperature, and seating.
2. Adjust any clutter or distractions.
3. Stand or sit in a relaxed, friendly way.
4. Greet the client warmly and observe their response.

Tips for Debriefing

- Ask the client for feedback on comfort levels.
- Notice if small changes in lighting or seat arrangement help them relax.

Troubleshooting Common Challenges

- If the room seems too cramped, remove extra furniture.
- If you appear stiff, do a quick posture check before sessions.

Reflection Questions

- How did changing the space affect the client's comfort?
- Did you see a difference in initial rapport?

Real-Life Example
Tony, 28, felt tense entering a dark office. His therapist later adjusted the lights and rearranged seating. At the next session, Tony reported feeling calmer right away.

Worksheet 2: Client Interests Exploration

The Purpose
You learn about the client's passions and daily life to show genuine care, establishing a relaxed flow of sharing.

The Rationale
Guntzviller et al. (2017) found that therapists who learn about a client's everyday interests build more trust and rapport early on.

Step-by-Step Instructions

1. Hand the client a brief questionnaire on hobbies or routines.
2. Ask follow-up questions (e.g., "What do you like about that hobby?").
3. Jot down key interests to revisit later.
4. Connect these interests to therapy goals when relevant.

Tips for Debriefing

- Emphasise your curiosity about their world.
- Reflect on surprising shared interests.

Troubleshooting Common Challenges

- If a client withholds details, offer gentle prompts.
- If they turn shy, reassure them you respect their privacy.

Reflection Questions

- How did hearing about their hobbies shape your sense of the client?
- Which interest could relate most to the therapy plan?

Real-Life Example
Ellen, 35, revealed she loves gardening. By discussing her favourite flowers early on, the therapist eased tension and found a shared topic to reference in future sessions.

Worksheet 3: Cultural and Contextual Inquiry

The Purpose
You open space for the client's cultural or community background. This fosters respect and a sense of safety.

The Rationale
Sue and Sue (2012) emphasise that understanding culture leads to better alignment with the client's worldview, increasing comfort and collaboration.

Step-by-Step Instructions

1. Invite the client to share cultural influences or traditions.
2. Listen carefully for language or norms that guide their decisions.
3. Check how these factors might affect therapy goals.
4. Discuss any adaptations you can make to honour their context.

Tips for Debriefing

- Ask how it felt to share these cultural elements.
- Acknowledge the importance of their traditions.

Troubleshooting Common Challenges

- If they're wary, remind them that their input shapes the therapy process.
- If unsure about certain customs, gently ask for clarification.

Reflection Questions

- Did learning about their background change your approach?
- How might cultural aspects impact treatment planning?

Real-Life Example
Lina, 40, mentioned extended family gatherings were common. Her therapist asked respectful questions on how these events shaped her daily stresses, leading to more nuanced support.

Worksheet 4: Icebreaker Open-Ended Questions

The Purpose
You create a comfortable launch to sessions by posing neutral, open-ended prompts that invite personal storytelling.

The Rationale
Miller and Rollnick (2013) note that open-ended starters help clients share thoughts freely, promoting deeper conversation early on.

Step-by-Step Instructions

1. Prepare a short list of general prompts (e.g., "What's been on your mind lately?").
2. Ask one or two at session start.
3. Maintain eye contact and an encouraging posture.
4. Follow their response with reflection or gentle prompts.

Tips for Debriefing

- Notice topics they quickly focus on.
- Let them lead the direction.

Troubleshooting Common Challenges

- If they seem hesitant, pick a simpler question.
- If they drift off topic, gently bring them back to a key theme.

Reflection Questions

- Which question led to the most engaged reply?
- Did you see any changes in the client's comfort?

Real-Life Example
Ed, 50, arrived looking uneasy. The therapist asked, "What recent event would you like me to know about?" Ed shared a family story, relaxing as the conversation flowed.

Worksheet 5: Identifying Best Communication Styles

The Purpose
You learn how the client prefers feedback and discussion, which prevents misunderstandings and fosters warmth.

The Rationale
A study in the Journal of Counselling Psychology (Brown & Woods, 2017) showed that when therapists tailor communication to clients' style, rapport increases quickly.

Step-by-Step Instructions

1. Ask the client how they like to receive supportive feedback.
2. Inquire about pace and detail they find most helpful.
3. Discuss any sensitivities (tone, language, or directness).
4. Keep notes to guide future sessions.

Tips for Debriefing

- Acknowledge their preferences, even if they differ from your usual style.
- Summarise key points to confirm you understood them.

Troubleshooting Common Challenges

- If they say "I'm not sure," suggest a few examples to spark ideas.
- If they test multiple styles, adapt session by session.

Reflection Questions

- How did clarifying their style change the session's tone?
- Did you feel more confident adjusting your delivery?

Real-Life Example
Paula, 28, said she prefers calm, step-by-step feedback. The therapist slowed down, offering short, clear guidance. Paula felt more valued and engaged.

Worksheet 6: Rapport Tracking Sheet

The Purpose
You record each session's comfort and openness levels to see what fosters better trust over time.

The Rationale
According to Gelso (2014), tracking rapport helps therapists notice patterns and refine their approach, leading to stronger outcomes.

Step-by-Step Instructions

1. Create a simple grid with columns for date, comfort score (1–10), and observations.
2. After the session, quickly jot down key impressions.
3. Highlight any events or topics that boosted or harmed rapport.
4. Revisit the sheet monthly to note trends.

Tips for Debriefing

- Share improvements or concerns with the client if it seems relevant.
- Use data to tweak your style or environment.

Troubleshooting Common Challenges

- If you forget to record details, set a brief reminder after each session.
- If no clear pattern emerges, try additional detail in your notes.

Reflection Questions

- Did you spot a boost in rapport after changing your approach?
- Which session had the highest comfort score, and why?

Real-Life Example
Diego, 38, felt anxious at first. Over six weeks, the therapist noted how calm language and a warmer greeting raised comfort scores from 4 to 7.

Worksheet 7: Reflective Listening Challenge

The Purpose
You dedicate a session to reflecting the client's words back, limiting advice. This boosts empathy and encourages deeper sharing.

The Rationale
Rogers (1957) found that clients feel more accepted and open when they hear their words reflected accurately, without judgement.

Step-by-Step Instructions

1. For one session, vow not to solve or correct.
2. Repeat or paraphrase the client's statements.
3. When they pause, say, "It sounds like you're feeling…"
4. Observe their reactions to your reflections.

Tips for Debriefing

- Check if the client felt more heard.
- Mention you temporarily avoided offering solutions.

Troubleshooting Common Challenges

- If they ask for advice, remind them you're listening deeply first.
- If you slip into solutions, notice it and return to reflection.

Reflection Questions

- How did focusing on reflections change the session's dynamic?
- Did the client elaborate more?

Real-Life Example
Ramona, 29, was used to quick tips. Hearing her own words reflected, she paused and shared more details. She later said she felt truly heard.

Worksheet 8: Empathic Statements Database

The Purpose
You gather meaningful phrases that capture concern and respect, ready to use when clients need reassurance.

The Rationale
Elliott et al. (2011) highlight that consistent empathic statements encourage clients to share vulnerable topics, helping therapy progress.

Step-by-Step Instructions

1. Compile a list of empathic lines (e.g., "I see how painful that is.").
2. Practise reciting them with sincere tone.
3. Document sessions to learn which phrases resonate with different clients.
4. Refine the database over time.

Tips for Debriefing

- Ask the client if any statement felt especially supportive.
- Stay natural, avoiding a robotic feel.

Troubleshooting Common Challenges

- If a phrase feels forced, adapt it to your own style.
- If the client reacts negatively, ask for clarity.

Reflection Questions

- Which new statement felt genuine?
- Did any statement spark a positive shift?

Real-Life Example
A list including "It sounds like that took a lot of courage" helped Nina, 42, feel proud discussing her first attempt at socialising after a long isolation.

Worksheet 9: Small Talk with Purpose

The Purpose
You use brief, friendly conversation at the session start to reduce anxiety and set a welcoming tone.

The Rationale
Kivlighan et al. (2019) found that a light rapport-building chat can calm client nerves, leading to smoother transitions into deeper subjects.

Step-by-Step Instructions

1. Greet the client with a simple question: "How was your journey here?"
2. Chat for one or two minutes about safe topics (weather, a public event).
3. Observe the client's response and comfort.
4. Gently shift toward therapy goals.

Tips for Debriefing

- Notice if they perk up or remain distant.
- Keep it short to avoid tangents.

Troubleshooting Common Challenges

- If they seem eager to start therapy topics, transition quickly.
- If they appear closed off, try simpler remarks.

Reflection Questions

- Did short small talk help them relax?
- How can you see this approach improving future sessions?

Real-Life Example
Andy, 31, was tense on arrival. A brief comment on the sunshine outside made him smile, reducing his tension before deeper questions started.

Worksheet 10: Shared Agenda Worksheet

The Purpose
You collaborate with the client to decide session goals, ensuring alignment and building shared ownership.

The Rationale
Miller and Rollnick (2013) demonstrate that a clear joint plan increases motivation and helps both parties stay on track.

Step-by-Step Instructions

1. Invite the client to suggest what they want to explore today.
2. Add your ideas or concerns as well.
3. List both sets on a single page.
4. Decide the order or priority together.

Tips for Debriefing

- Confirm that the client feels heard in forming the plan.
- Revisit it halfway through to check progress.

Troubleshooting Common Challenges

- If they say "I don't know," propose a quick brainstorming approach.
- If time runs short, clarify what can wait until next session.

Reflection Questions

- Did the shared plan help the client feel more involved?
- What shifted once you agreed on mutual targets?

Real-Life Example
Gina, 27, arrived unsure of her focus. After brainstorming, she and her therapist prioritised stress at work. They finished the session feeling a united sense of purpose.

Worksheet 11: Vocal Tone Awareness

The Purpose
You monitor how your voice's pitch and warmth can affect trust, ensuring you project a compassionate tone.

The Rationale
Paralinguistic research (Burgoon et al., 2016) shows that supportive tone fosters positive rapport, making clients more relaxed.

Step-by-Step Instructions

1. Record a short segment of your session.
2. Listen for moments when your voice might sound tense or distant.
3. Practise speaking at a softer volume, with pauses.
4. Compare your approach in the next session.

Tips for Debriefing

- Check with the client about how your voice impacted their comfort.
- Keep notes on any improvements you notice.

Troubleshooting Common Challenges

- If your voice is naturally loud, take deeper, slower breaths before speaking.
- If you feel nervous, warm up with a calm breathing routine.

Reflection Questions

- Did altering your tone shift the client's manner of sharing?
- Which vocal habits need the most attention?

Real-Life Example
Becca, a therapist, reviewed her recordings and realised she often sounded brisk when stressed. Lowering her pitch and speaking calmly helped her clients open up more.

Worksheet 12: Recognising Client Strengths Early

The Purpose
You offer positive feedback about the client's unique qualities from the start, boosting their sense of acceptance.

The Rationale
Seligman and Csikszentmihalyi (2000) highlight that early recognition of strengths fosters hope and resilience in therapy.

Step-by-Step Instructions

1. In the first session, note at least one strength (e.g., determination).
2. Gently point it out: "I appreciate how thorough you are in describing details."
3. Ask how they feel hearing that.
4. Document these strengths for future reference.

Tips for Debriefing

- Remind clients their positive traits form a foundation for progress.
- See if they agree with your observations or have others to add.

Troubleshooting Common Challenges

- If they brush off compliments, acknowledge it may feel unusual.
- If it's hard to find strengths, look for small efforts or attitudes.

Reflection Questions

- Did the client brighten up when strengths were noted?
- What difference did this make in building trust?

Real-Life Example
During their initial meeting, Tamika, 34, was praised for her insightful observations. She admitted she rarely heard such affirmations and felt encouraged to keep talking.

Worksheet 13: Boundaries and Safety

The Purpose
You clarify guidelines, confidentiality, and mutual respect. This ensures a consistent, protected environment for therapy.

The Rationale
Barnett et al. (2007) report that when boundaries are clear, clients feel safer revealing sensitive information.

Step-by-Step Instructions

1. Explain confidentiality limits (e.g., risk of harm).
2. State your availability (e.g., contact outside sessions).
3. Discuss respect for each other's time and boundaries.
4. Invite any questions about these guidelines.

Tips for Debriefing

- Ask if the client feels relieved or cautious regarding these rules.
- Reassure them that clarity prevents confusion later.

Troubleshooting Common Challenges

- If they seem uneasy, carefully revisit any clause that worries them.
- If they request more flexibility, see where compromise can be made safely.

Reflection Questions

- Did establishing boundaries help the client relax?
- Which guideline felt most important to them?

Real-Life Example
Rose, 29, asked if she could email between sessions. Her therapist explained time limitations while affirming willingness to read short updates. Rose found comfort in having a clear plan.

Worksheet 14: Personalising Goals

The Purpose
You invite the client to define success on their own terms. This encourages ownership and motivation.

The Rationale
Sheldon and Kasser (1998) show that when goals match personal values, engagement increases and clients often sustain effort longer.

Step-by-Step Instructions

1. Ask the client what positive change they'd like to see.
2. Encourage specifics: "What does success look like for you?"
3. Note the emotional meaning behind each goal.
4. Summarise their targets in their own words.

Tips for Debriefing

- Verify you heard them correctly.
- Link smaller steps to the bigger outcome they envision.

Troubleshooting Common Challenges

- If they give vague answers, gently prompt for clarity.
- If the goal is very broad, help them break it into a shorter-term milestone.

Reflection Questions

- How does defining success in personal terms feel?
- Which goal resonates most strongly with them right now?

Real-Life Example
Daniel, 37, decided success meant fewer panic attacks and a calmer workday. The therapist wrote these aims in Daniel's words, making the direction more concrete.

Worksheet 15: Reflecting on Common Ground

The Purpose
You identify shared experiences or interests with the client, creating a sense of partnership and human connection.

The Rationale
Norcross and Lambert (2018) show that noticing overlaps in experiences can lower perceived hierarchy and foster closeness.

Step-by-Step Instructions

1. Listen for any mention of interests you share (e.g., a sport, a local event).
2. Briefly acknowledge that similarity ("I'm also a fan of that team.").
3. Let the client lead if they want to discuss it further.
4. Keep the focus on them, but gently weave in that small connection.

Tips for Debriefing

- Emphasise that even small similarities can ease tension.
- Remain sincere and avoid fake bonding.

Troubleshooting Common Challenges

- If you have no real overlap, don't invent one.
- If the client looks uncomfortable, respect boundaries.

Reflection Questions

- Did pointing out common ground shift the atmosphere?
- How can you balance shared experiences with professional roles?

Real-Life Example
Joe, 40, mentioned volunteering at an animal shelter. His therapist kindly shared she once volunteered too. Joe felt more comfortable, seeing her as relatable.

Worksheet 16: Using Metaphors

The Purpose
You employ a metaphor that resonates with the client's interests to simplify complex ideas and strengthen rapport.

The Rationale
Tay et al. (2018) found that well-chosen metaphors bridge understanding, especially when drawn from the client's personal interests.

Step-by-Step Instructions

1. Ask about their hobbies or passions (sports, music, cooking).
2. Craft a parallel that links therapy progress to that activity.
3. Use the metaphor during challenging discussions.
4. Check if it feels meaningful to them.

Tips for Debriefing

- Confirm that the metaphor captures their reality.
- Adjust if they find it confusing or irrelevant.

Troubleshooting Common Challenges

- If you pick a metaphor unrelated to them, it falls flat.
- If the metaphor feels forced, collaborate on a better one.

Reflection Questions

- How does imagining therapy through this metaphor help them see solutions?
- Did they feel more engaged?

Real-Life Example
A client who loves cooking compared her emotional work to refining a recipe. She saw each small step as adding "ingredients" to improve her outcomes.

Worksheet 17: Eliciting Client Insights

The Purpose
You highlight the client's own reflections on their process or progress, showing respect for their expertise in themselves.

The Rationale
Cooper and McLeod (2011) found that inviting clients to evaluate therapy fosters empowerment and encourages deeper self-knowledge.

Step-by-Step Instructions

1. At session midpoint, ask, "What have you realised about yourself this week?"
2. Listen closely, reflect, and gently prod for more details.
3. Encourage them to link these insights to their goals.
4. Take note for later reference.

Tips for Debriefing

- Thank them for their perspective.
- Reinforce that their observations are valuable to shaping therapy.

Troubleshooting Common Challenges

- If they struggle, ask about small shifts or thoughts since the last meeting.
- If they downplay their insight, affirm that even minor observations matter.

Reflection Questions

- Did exploring their own insights increase motivation?
- Which new discovery seemed most useful?

Real-Life Example
Brianna, 25, realised she felt calmer after a morning walk. Sharing this helped her see she could use walks to manage stress.

Worksheet 18: Non-Judgmental Curiosity

The Purpose
You practise staying curious rather than slipping into judgement or bias. This keeps the client comfortable expressing themselves.

The Rationale
Linehan (1993) stresses that curiosity without judgement fosters openness and helps clients reveal true concerns.

Step-by-Step Instructions

1. Use a personal checklist of mindful reminders (e.g., "Stay open," "Pause before reacting").
2. Notice any internal urges to correct or criticise.
3. Replace them with a question: "Can you tell me more about that?"
4. Continue the session while watching your own stance.

Tips for Debriefing

- Evaluate how it felt to hold back judgement.
- Discuss with a colleague if you find certain triggers.

Troubleshooting Common Challenges

- If you catch yourself being critical, gently refocus.
- If the client expects judgement, reassure them they're safe here.

Reflection Questions

- Did the client speak more freely when you stayed curious?
- Which prompt helped you remain open-minded?

Real-Life Example
Austin, 32, shared a behaviour he feared others would judge. The therapist's calm questions showed acceptance, allowing Austin to reveal deeper worries without shame.

Worksheet 19: Common Pitfalls in Rapport Building

The Purpose
You identify frequent pitfalls like interrupting or rushing, then plan to avoid them to preserve trust.

The Rationale
Swift et al. (2017) argue that being aware of typical therapist missteps (e.g., talking too much) reduces client dropout and enhances engagement.

Step-by-Step Instructions

1. List common rapport blunders: cutting off the client, offering forced solutions, using jargon.
2. Mark which ones you've done.
3. Write a brief plan to correct each.
4. Keep the list visible during sessions as a reminder.

Tips for Debriefing

- Share your plan with a supervisor or peer for feedback.
- Check in regularly to see if these pitfalls reduce.

Troubleshooting Common Challenges

- If you slip up, apologise briefly and refocus on the client's voice.
- If you feel rushed, schedule more time for sessions.

Reflection Questions

- Which pitfall affects you the most?
- How have clients reacted when those mistakes happen?

Real-Life Example
Jared, a counsellor, noticed he often interrupted. By tracking it, he cut back on interruptions, and his clients began speaking more openly.

Worksheet 20: Practice of Genuine Compliments

The Purpose
You learn to offer heartfelt praise instead of empty flattery, helping clients feel valued for real attributes or efforts.

The Rationale
According to Biswas-Diener (2010), specific, authentic compliments encourage self-esteem and deeper trust.

Step-by-Step Instructions

1. Think of a concrete quality or achievement you observe (e.g., perseverance).
2. Express it plainly ("I appreciate how you kept going despite challenges.").
3. Watch the client's reaction.
4. Avoid overdoing it; pick one sincere compliment per session.

Tips for Debriefing

- Ask if the client felt supported by the compliment.
- Encourage them to take ownership of that positive trait.

Troubleshooting Common Challenges

- If they dismiss it, affirm you mean it sincerely.
- If you can't find something to praise, look for even small steps or attempts.

Reflection Questions

- Did the client appear more open after hearing genuine praise?
- How did it feel offering carefully chosen compliments?

Real-Life Example
Carla, 39, rarely accepted praise. Hearing, "You showed true dedication in writing that journal entry," made her smile and share more about her growth.

Worksheet 21: Calming Presence Routine

The Purpose
You centre yourself before each session through a quick mindfulness check, ensuring you enter the room with a calm, reassuring energy.

The Rationale
Kabat-Zinn (1990) indicates that therapists who ground themselves can transmit calmness, improving rapport and trust.

Step-by-Step Instructions

1. Pause for one minute before the client arrives.
2. Close your eyes and focus on gentle breathing.
3. Release tension in your shoulders and jaw.
4. Enter the session with a calm mindset.

Tips for Debriefing

- Notice if this practice lowered your stress.
- Ask the client if they perceived a calmer atmosphere.

Troubleshooting Common Challenges

- If you feel rushed, try a shorter version of the routine.
- If your mind wanders, gently refocus on breathing.

Reflection Questions

- Did this quick pause help you feel more present?
- How did it affect the flow of conversation?

Real-Life Example
Before meeting a high-anxiety client, Sarah, a therapist, used this one-minute calming pause. She felt more balanced, and the client sensed her steady tone.

Worksheet 22: Supporting Self-Exploration

The Purpose
You spark the client's introspection by using subtle prompts that invite them to find their own answers.

The Rationale
Cooper (2008) showed that encouraging self-reflection increases a client's sense of ownership, building stronger rapport and lasting change.

Step-by-Step Instructions

1. Offer a gentle question: "How do you interpret that feeling?"
2. Pause, letting them reflect without interruption.
3. Validate their emerging thoughts.
4. Encourage them to write or journal after the session.

Tips for Debriefing

- Reinforce that they are the main source of wisdom about themselves.
- Note any breakthroughs that come from quiet reflection.

Troubleshooting Common Challenges

- If they resist, frame it as an invitation, not pressure.
- If they ask for your opinion, echo their thoughts first.

Reflection Questions

- Did you see them reach a new understanding?
- How might they build on this insight outside sessions?

Real-Life Example
Carl, 37, rarely paused to reflect. By asking him to interpret his stress signals, the therapist watched him connect the dots about his overwork and self-criticism.

Worksheet 23: Open vs. Closed Questions Audit

The Purpose
You track how many open and closed questions you ask, aiming to expand open questions for deeper client engagement.

The Rationale
According to Miller and Rollnick (2013), open questions promote exploration, while closed questions can limit discussion.

Step-by-Step Instructions

1. Record each question you ask during one session.
2. Label them as open (invites elaborate replies) or closed (yes/no).
3. Tally results.
4. Aim to boost open questions in the next session.

Tips for Debriefing

- Discuss with a peer or supervisor your tallies.
- Practise rephrasing closed questions in a more open style.

Troubleshooting Common Challenges

- If you default to closed questions under stress, keep notes on a sticky pad to remind yourself.
- If the session topic needs specifics, use open follow-ups.

Reflection Questions

- Were you surprised by the ratio of open to closed?
- How did the client respond differently to each type?

Real-Life Example
Mel, a counsellor, found she used 12 closed and 5 open questions in one session. After adjusting, she asked 10 open ones next time, improving the flow of conversation.

Worksheet 24: Affirmation Checklist

The Purpose
You plan purposeful affirmations about the client's resilience, creativity, or kindness. This encourages them to see their own worth.

The Rationale
Maddux (2002) indicates that targeted affirmation can boost self-belief, reinforcing positive steps the client takes.

Step-by-Step Instructions

1. List qualities you notice (e.g., problem-solving skill, empathy).
2. Write a short statement for each: "I see you're very resourceful."
3. Check them off after using them in session.
4. Observe how each affirmation influences the dialogue.

Tips for Debriefing

- Confirm the client felt the affirmation was genuine.
- Let them add qualities they identify in themselves.

Troubleshooting Common Challenges

- If they dismiss it, gently reiterate examples that support the affirmation.
- If you run out of ideas, reflect on past sessions for hidden strengths.

Reflection Questions

- Which affirmation sparked the biggest response?
- How do you plan to build on their stated strengths?

Real-Life Example
Tim, 44, always saw himself as "lazy." Hearing his therapist affirm his consistent attendance and small achievements helped him redefine himself as reliable.

Worksheet 25: Attention to Non-Verbal Cues

The Purpose
You sharpen your awareness of physical signals like posture, eye contact, or fidgeting, adapting your approach to the client's comfort.

The Rationale
Mehrabian's (1972) findings indicate that non-verbal messages often convey more than words, shaping rapport strongly.

Step-by-Step Instructions

1. In each session, note if the client fidgets, avoids eye contact, or looks relaxed.
2. Gently acknowledge if you see tension (e.g., "I notice you're clenching your hands.").
3. Ask if they want to pause or if something is uneasy.
4. Adjust your tone and posture to match the client's comfort zone.

Tips for Debriefing

- Check if your observation felt supportive, not intrusive.
- Track how non-verbal cues shift throughout the session.

Troubleshooting Common Challenges

- If the client becomes self-conscious, reassure them you aim to understand.
- If you misread a cue, allow them to clarify.

Reflection Questions

- Did observing body language lead to new insights?
- How might you refine this skill further?

Real-Life Example
Beth, 33, tapped her foot whenever she discussed her mother. The therapist gently named it, leading Beth to realise she got anxious at that topic.

Worksheet 26: Mirroring Energy Levels

The Purpose
You notice the client's emotional tone or energy and match it. This shows respect for their current state, helping them feel understood.

The Rationale
Research by Koole and Tschacher (2016) shows that subtle mirroring can increase empathy and synchrony in therapeutic relationships.

Step-by-Step Instructions

1. Assess if the client is subdued, animated, or tense.
2. Modulate your voice pace and volume slightly toward their level.
3. As they relax or brighten, gently match that shift.
4. Avoid imitating them too closely. Keep it natural.

Tips for Debriefing

- See if they commented or seemed more connected.
- Remain genuine: don't mimic, just align.

Troubleshooting Common Challenges

- If they're very high-energy, keep calm while acknowledging their enthusiasm.
- If they're depressed, avoid matching gloom too heavily—aim for gentle warmth.

Reflection Questions

- Did mirroring their energy help them open up?
- How did you maintain authenticity?

Real-Life Example
Luis, 19, spoke quickly, full of excitement. His therapist sped up her speech slightly. He noticed the therapist's engagement and felt comfortable sharing even more.

Worksheet 27: Highlighting Common Goals

The Purpose
You show that you share the client's aim for growth. This fosters a sense of teamwork in the therapeutic process.

The Rationale
Lambert (2013) notes that clarifying mutual purpose increases collaboration, making clients feel supported and validated.

Step-by-Step Instructions

1. Ask the client for their main aim.
2. Express your eagerness to support that aim.
3. Find at least one overlap between your approach and their desired outcome.
4. State it clearly: "We both want to help you manage stress better."

Tips for Debriefing

- Re-check if the client truly resonates with that shared goal.
- Use inclusive language ("We," "together").

Troubleshooting Common Challenges

- If they distrust professionals, emphasise the mutual nature of the work.
- If their goal shifts, revisit and form a new shared vision.

Reflection Questions

- Does naming shared goals improve the client's sense of direction?
- How can you refer back to this shared purpose in future sessions?

Real-Life Example
Ellie, 23, admitted she wanted better anxiety management. The therapist stated, "I'm here to help you feel calmer day to day. We're on the same side." Ellie smiled at the unity.

Worksheet 28: Story Sharing

The Purpose
You invite the client to tell a brief personal anecdote, then respond with supportive reflections to deepen rapport.

The Rationale
Maruna (2001) suggests that sharing personal stories helps clients make sense of experiences and feel known, increasing trust.

Step-by-Step Instructions

1. Request a short narrative: "Could you tell me about a time you felt proud?"
2. Stay attentive, nodding or jotting notes.
3. Reflect back an emotional element you hear.
4. Thank them for sharing.

Tips for Debriefing

- Focus on how the story shaped their feelings.
- Encourage them to reflect on what the story might reveal about their resilience.

Troubleshooting Common Challenges

- If they go on tangents, gently guide them to the main points.
- If they share something traumatic, switch to a supportive stance, validating their courage.

Reflection Questions

- Did you notice any key themes in their story?
- How can this anecdote inform therapy goals?

Real-Life Example
Miguel, 45, described learning guitar as a teen and realising he could master new skills. The therapist highlighted his perseverance, boosting his current self-confidence.

Worksheet 29: Language Pace Analysis

The Purpose
You record your session to examine the speed of your speech versus the client's. Adjusting pace can improve comfort and rapport.

The Rationale
Gallagher and Vella-Brodrick (2008) show that pacing speech to match the client's rhythm can create a smoother connection.

Step-by-Step Instructions

1. Record a brief part of the session.
2. Notice if you're speaking faster or slower than them.
3. Practise matching their tempo during a follow-up exchange.
4. Compare the difference in engagement.

Tips for Debriefing

- Mention if they felt more at ease when the pace was closer.
- Adjust if they speak extremely fast or slow.

Troubleshooting Common Challenges

- If you naturally talk very fast, remind yourself to breathe and pause.
- If they talk slowly, stay patient rather than rushing them.

Reflection Questions

- Did mirroring speed help them open up more fluidly?
- How might pacing reduce miscommunication?

Real-Life Example
Chris, 40, spoke slowly due to anxiety. The therapist recorded the session, then consciously slowed their own rate next time. Chris felt less pressured and shared more details.

Worksheet 30: Elicit 'What Matters to You?'

The Purpose
You uncover the client's core values or priorities early on, anchoring therapy in their deepest motivations.

The Rationale
Ryan and Deci (2000) stress that autonomy and personal meaning drive engagement. Knowing what truly counts for the client fosters trust and clarity.

Step-by-Step Instructions

1. Ask, "What is most important to you in life right now?"
2. Listen, reflecting any strong emotions.
3. Explore how therapy can support those priorities.
4. Keep these responses in mind when setting goals.

Tips for Debriefing

- Validate their choices, even if unusual or unexpected.
- Remind them that therapy aligns with these core wishes.

Troubleshooting Common Challenges

- If they struggle, prompt ideas like health, family, faith, career.
- If they pick many, help them focus on the top one or two.

Reflection Questions

- How does discussing personal values deepen trust?
- Did you see the client's motivation brighten?

Real-Life Example
Hannah, 32, declared family stability as her main focus. Connecting each therapy step to that value kept her energised, increasing her commitment to the process.

Worksheet 31: Offering Choices

The Purpose
You let clients pick from possible tasks or focuses, reinforcing their autonomy and comfort in the therapeutic setting.

The Rationale
Deci and Ryan (2008) point out that having options boosts intrinsic motivation and fosters a sense of safety in therapy.

Step-by-Step Instructions

1. Present two or three possible activities ("We could explore your anxiety triggers or review last week's progress.").
2. Ask the client which they'd prefer first.
3. Follow their lead while remaining prepared to adapt.
4. Note how they respond to taking the lead.

Tips for Debriefing

- Emphasise they have the right to decide what feels most helpful.
- If they're hesitant, gently encourage them to try picking one.

Troubleshooting Common Challenges

- If they always say "You decide," offer a small push for them to choose.
- If they can't choose, use a quick pro/con discussion for each option.

Reflection Questions

- Did the client show more engagement after selecting a path?
- How might repeated choice-giving strengthen rapport?

Real-Life Example
Roy, 41, had trouble trusting experts. Being offered a choice of topics each session soothed him, proving that his voice mattered.

Worksheet 32: Reflecting Personal Responsibility

The Purpose
You encourage clients to recognise their role in decisions or progress, highlighting their power to initiate change.

The Rationale
According to Miller and Rollnick (2013), guiding clients to own their actions fosters a sense of control and positive momentum in therapy.

Step-by-Step Instructions

1. When discussing a challenge, paraphrase with a focus on their choices: "You decided to do this…"
2. Invite them to confirm or elaborate.
3. Ask how this sense of responsibility feels.
4. Link it to potential steps forward.

Tips for Debriefing

- Reinforce that acknowledging responsibility doesn't mean self-blame.
- Praise them for each brave admission of personal agency.

Troubleshooting Common Challenges

- If they deflect blame, gently show evidence of their involvement in outcomes.
- If they feel guilty, balance it with empathy and solutions.

Reflection Questions

- Did noticing their agency spark more willingness to act?
- How can you keep reinforcing this idea without overwhelming them?

Real-Life Example
Caleb, 30, blamed others for his anger issues. Hearing the therapist reflect, "You chose to respond by walking away," helped him realise he had options, increasing hope.

Worksheet 33: Visual Representation of Rapport

The Purpose
You invite the client to draw or symbolise how they currently feel about the therapy relationship, revealing hidden comfort or tension.

The Rationale
Hinz (2009) found that creative exercises help clients communicate subtle emotions. Visual methods can uncover helpful insights into rapport quality.

Step-by-Step Instructions

1. Offer paper and markers.
2. Ask them to sketch or use shapes/colours that represent their comfort level.
3. Encourage them to label or briefly explain the image.
4. Explore any interesting elements or themes.

Tips for Debriefing

- Listen without judgement.
- Avoid over-interpreting; let them explain meaning first.

Troubleshooting Common Challenges

- If they resist drawing, invite them to choose words or metaphors instead.
- If the image is unclear, gently ask clarifying questions.

Reflection Questions

- Did the process reveal any hidden tension or trust?
- How can you adjust your approach based on this?

Real-Life Example
A teen client drew two figures on a wide bridge, indicating she felt somewhat close to her therapist but still cautious. This led to a talk about building deeper trust.

Worksheet 34: Transitions with Care

The Purpose
You manage the shift from light talk to deeper issues smoothly, reducing abrupt changes that might jolt or unsettle the client.

The Rationale
Wachtel (2011) explains that gentle transitions maintain safety, preventing clients from feeling caught off-guard when heavier topics arise.

Step-by-Step Instructions

1. Acknowledge the current topic: "We've chatted about your day."
2. Signal a shift: "Could we take a moment to explore that challenge you mentioned?"
3. Check if they feel ready.
4. Proceed once they confirm readiness.

Tips for Debriefing

- Reinforce that they can pause if it becomes uncomfortable.
- Validate any anxiety around deeper discussions.

Troubleshooting Common Challenges

- If they avoid big subjects, offer a gentle invitation instead of a push.
- If time is short, note it and plan to revisit next session.

Reflection Questions

- Did a careful transition make them more receptive?
- How can you refine your approach to serious topics?

Real-Life Example
Tina, 25, felt startled when previous counsellors jumped straight to trauma. By calmly asking if they could shift gears, her new therapist saw Tina relax and willingly go deeper.

Worksheet 35: Clarity of Roles

The Purpose
You define your duties and scope as a therapist while inviting the client to outline what they expect, creating an equal partnership.

The Rationale
Karver et al. (2006) note that transparent role discussion helps prevent misinterpretation and fosters a supportive alliance.

Step-by-Step Instructions

1. Briefly describe your role: listening, guiding, maintaining boundaries.
2. Ask, "What do you expect from me, and what responsibilities do you see for yourself?"
3. Discuss any mismatched expectations.
4. Summarise final role agreements.

Tips for Debriefing

- Revisit roles if confusion arises.
- Encourage the client to voice changes if they want more or less direction.

Troubleshooting Common Challenges

- If they treat you as a friend, clarify professional boundaries.
- If they want you to fix everything, emphasise shared effort.

Reflection Questions

- Did clarifying roles reduce confusion?
- How might you remind them of these roles if tensions occur?

Real-Life Example
During an early session, Omar asked if the therapist would solve his relationship

issues. After clarifying collaborative roles, Omar understood he'd be active in finding solutions.

Worksheet 36: Cross-Cultural Curiosity

The Purpose
You show open interest in traditions, beliefs, or practices that guide the client's decisions, promoting mutual respect.

The Rationale
Leong and Lee (2006) emphasise that sincere questions about culture help break down barriers and promote understanding.

Step-by-Step Instructions

1. Politely ask if the client's heritage or traditions influence their current situation.
2. Listen for details about family, community, or spiritual customs.
3. Show empathy through reflections ("That celebration sounds meaningful.").
4. Adjust therapy strategies if needed.

Tips for Debriefing

- Ask the client how they felt sharing cultural details.
- Affirm your respect for their background.

Troubleshooting Common Challenges

- If they are cautious, show genuine listening and no judgement.
- If you're unsure of a cultural reference, kindly request clarity.

Reflection Questions

- Did exploring culture strengthen trust?
- Which aspect of their background might shape therapy the most?

Real-Life Example

Samira, 45, explained a holiday ritual that helps her cope with stress. The therapist respectfully asked more about it, helping Samira feel proud and validated.

Worksheet 37: Envisioning Positive Outcomes

The Purpose

You encourage the client to imagine what a helpful therapeutic experience looks like, guiding both of you toward that vision.

The Rationale

Bandura (1997) suggests that picturing successful outcomes can boost confidence in achieving meaningful progress.

Step-by-Step Instructions

1. Invite the client to visualise a future session where they feel real progress.
2. Ask what changed in their life or mindset.
3. Reflect: "How could we work toward that outcome?"
4. Make a brief plan linking that vision to actual steps.

Tips for Debriefing

- Praise their ability to imagine a brighter scenario.
- Connect the vision to concrete actions now.

Troubleshooting Common Challenges

- If they only see negatives, gently help them consider one small positive shift.
- If they struggle to visualise, ask for any desired improvement, no matter how small.

Reflection Questions

- Did this forward-looking perspective energise them?
- How might you keep referring back to that image?

Real-Life Example
Derek, 29, pictured feeling calmer in social settings. The therapist asked what that calm scene might look like and used it as a motivation throughout therapy.

Worksheet 38: Using Touchstones

The Purpose
You and the client agree on a simple phrase or symbol that reminds both of you to stay on track when sessions drift.

The Rationale
Safran and Muran (2000) highlight that agreed-upon reminders can refocus conversation, preserving coherence and rapport.

Step-by-Step Instructions

1. Collaborate on a short phrase (e.g., "Check-in moment").
2. Decide that either one can say it if the discussion wanders.
3. Practise using it in session.
4. Evaluate if it brings you back to key themes.

Tips for Debriefing

- Ask if the client found it helpful or distracting.
- Adjust the phrase for comfort and practicality.

Troubleshooting Common Challenges

- If it's not used, gently remind the client it's available.
- If the phrase feels awkward, find a better one.

Reflection Questions

- Did using the touchstone phrase keep you on course?
- Would a different word or signal suit them better?

Real-Life Example
Julie, 33, and her therapist used "Pause Point." Whenever they rambled or felt lost, one said "Pause Point" and they regrouped, protecting session focus.

Worksheet 39: Checking Personal Biases

The Purpose
You reflect on your own assumptions or biases before each session, aiming to keep them from interfering with genuine rapport.

The Rationale
Ridley (2005) indicates that therapists who self-monitor their biases offer more balanced, client-centred care.

Step-by-Step Instructions

1. Note any immediate judgments you might hold (e.g., about a behaviour).
2. Ask yourself how these might colour your reactions.
3. Write a short intention: "I will keep an open mind about…"
4. Revisit this note post-session, evaluating your success.

Tips for Debriefing

- If a bias appeared mid-session, reflect on how you managed it.
- Seek supervision if certain biases repeatedly arise.

Troubleshooting Common Challenges

- If you catch yourself acting on bias, apologise to the client if needed and readjust.
- If biases are deeply rooted, consider further training.

Reflection Questions

- Did acknowledging bias change how you listened?
- How can you build a consistent habit of checking bias?

Real-Life Example
A therapist felt sceptical about a client's repeated job changes. After writing it down, she approached the session with open questions instead of assumptions, improving rapport.

Worksheet 40: Summarising for Rapport

The Purpose
You close each session with a concise recap, showing that you listened, understood, and value the client's input.

The Rationale
Miller and Rollnick (2013) observe that summarising validates client experiences and helps them feel affirmed.

Step-by-Step Instructions

1. Near the session's end, briefly highlight the main topics discussed.
2. Include key emotional tones and client insights.
3. Ask if the client agrees with or wants to amend the summary.
4. Confirm next steps or goals together.

Tips for Debriefing

- Encourage them to share if anything was missed or misheard.
- Note any new areas to explore next time.

Troubleshooting Common Challenges

- If you rush, you may omit essential points. Allocate a few minutes for the summary.
- If the client is silent, gently prompt them for feedback on accuracy.

Reflection Questions

- Did a clear closing summary boost the client's sense of being heard?

- What might you adjust in your summarising style?

Real-Life Example
Marla, 24, appreciated hearing the therapist recount her main struggle (sleep anxiety) and highlight her plan to try a breathing technique before bedtime. She left feeling understood and prepared.

With these 40 worksheets, you can refine the process of creating comfort, trust, and genuine connection in every session. By staying consistent and thoughtful in your approach to rapport-building, you help clients feel safe enough to share, explore, and move forward.

Focusing and Setting the Agenda

Worksheets in this group help clarify what the client truly wants to address. They encourage identifying priorities and establishing a clear direction for sessions. By honing in on specific goals or issues, you keep the process structured and ensure that you and the client share a defined path forward.

Worksheet 1: Goal Brainstorm

Title
Goal Brainstorm

The Purpose
You help the client gather every area of concern or change they want. This encourages free-flowing ideas before picking key priorities.

The Rationale
Prochaska and DiClemente (1983) suggest that identifying multiple issues early allows a more deliberate choice of focus. Listing all possibilities helps clients avoid missing hidden needs.

Step-by-Step Instructions

1. Invite the client to jot down every issue or aspiration they have.
2. Encourage them not to filter or rank at first.
3. After the list is complete, read it together.
4. Ask which items feel most pressing or achievable.

Tips for Debriefing

- Affirm that no goal is "too small" or "too big."
- Notice if the client hesitates to mention certain items.

Troubleshooting Common Challenges

- If the client struggles, prompt them with broad life areas (health, relationships, etc.).
- If the list is long, summarise as you go to maintain clarity.

Reflection Questions

- Which item on your list sparks the most energy or emotion?
- Did writing them down offer any relief or insight?

Real-Life Example
Nina wrote down "improve finances, reduce stress, move to a new flat." She felt relieved seeing her worries in one place, realising they overlapped in ways she hadn't noticed.

Worksheet 2: Prioritisation Grid

Title
Prioritisation Grid

The Purpose
You weigh urgency against importance, allowing the client to see which issues demand immediate attention and which can wait.

The Rationale
Moran (2015) explains that a clear matrix (urgent vs. important) helps clients focus energy on tasks that truly matter, avoiding wasted effort.

Step-by-Step Instructions

1. Draw a 2x2 grid. Label rows "Urgent" and "Not Urgent," columns "Important" and "Less Important."
2. Sort each item from the goal list into one of the four boxes.
3. Discuss which box seems biggest or most critical.
4. Decide which issues the client wants to tackle first.

Tips for Debriefing

- Check how the client feels about postponing less urgent tasks.
- Stress that some issues can still be monitored even if not top priority now.

Troubleshooting Common Challenges

- If they resist ranking, remind them this is a temporary tool.
- If they label everything as urgent and important, help them identify at least one area that might be less critical.

Reflection Questions

- Did the grid reveal any surprises about urgency vs. importance?
- How will you address tasks in the top priority quadrant?

Real-Life Example
Ethan placed "finding a new job" in urgent and important. "Learning piano" went to not urgent but important. This clarity helped him schedule time to job hunt first.

Worksheet 3: Core Issues Identification

Title
Core Issues Identification

The Purpose
You help the client dig below surface problems, distinguishing the deeper drivers from symptoms.

The Rationale
Miller and Rollnick (2013) highlight that exploring root causes ensures therapy targets the actual source, preventing superficial fixes.

Step-by-Step Instructions

1. Have the client pick one pressing concern.
2. Ask "What might lie beneath this problem?"
3. Gently keep asking "What else could be fuelling it?" until you find a deeper theme.
4. Summarise the root issue in their words.

Tips for Debriefing

- Emphasise that identifying deeper causes can spark lasting solutions.
- Keep your questions calm and open-ended.

Troubleshooting Common Challenges

- If the client struggles, reflect potential patterns from previous sessions.
- If they feel uncomfortable, proceed more slowly, respecting their pace.

Reflection Questions

- Did uncovering root causes shift your view of the problem?
- Which insight felt most eye-opening?

Real-Life Example
Maria said her main issue was procrastinating at work, but repeated questions revealed fear of failure from childhood expectations.

Worksheet 4: Agenda Mapping

Title
Agenda Mapping

The Purpose
You develop a visual outline of multiple topics or goals so the client can see how they interconnect.

The Rationale
According to Knight (2009), mapping out issues fosters clarity and reduces overwhelm. Seeing a bigger picture allows strategic decisions about which path to follow first.

Step-by-Step Instructions

1. Draw a central circle with the client's name or main theme.
2. Branch out smaller circles for each topic they want to discuss.
3. Label or colour-code related topics.
4. Ask which branch is the best starting point.

Tips for Debriefing

- Notice if the client sees any surprising links.

- Encourage them to pick one or two branches to tackle in the next session.

Troubleshooting Common Challenges

- If they have too many branches, group smaller ones together under a broader heading.
- If the client is not visual, consider a short bullet list approach.

Reflection Questions

- Did connecting issues help you notice overlapping patterns?
- How did you feel deciding which branch to explore first?

Real-Life Example
Arjun drew circles for "family conflict," "anxiety," "financial debt," and realised "family conflict" triggered anxiety, making debt management harder.

Worksheet 5: Value-Based Focusing

Title
Value-Based Focusing

The Purpose
You tie each potential topic to the client's core principles (family, health, authenticity) so they see why an issue matters on a deeper level.

The Rationale
Sheldon and Kasser (1998) found that linking therapy goals to personal values boosts commitment and satisfaction with progress.

Step-by-Step Instructions

1. Ask the client to pick one main value (e.g., "family").
2. Review each goal or issue, connecting it back to this value: "How does this goal align with your family focus?"
3. Repeat for any other values they hold.

4. Mark which goals strongly reflect each value.

Tips for Debriefing

- Reinforce that aligning with values can spark motivation.
- Encourage them to note any emotional response during the process.

Troubleshooting Common Challenges

- If they're unsure of their values, revisit a values clarification worksheet.
- If a goal doesn't fit a value, explore if it's truly important or can be reframed.

Reflection Questions

- How does linking a goal to your values affect your drive to pursue it?
- Which value felt most powerful today?

Real-Life Example
Jenny cherished "community." Realising that managing her social anxiety would help her join local volunteer groups, she grew more determined to address it.

Worksheet 6: Readiness Assessment

Title
Readiness Assessment

The Purpose
You measure if the client feels prepared to address each item on their list, preventing rushed or forced attempts that might fail.

The Rationale
Rollnick and Allison (2004) suggest that gauging readiness with a simple scale (1–10) informs the therapist about a client's willingness and motivation, guiding better pacing.

Step-by-Step Instructions

1. List each potential goal or issue.
2. Ask the client to rate their readiness on a 1–10 scale.
3. Discuss why they picked that number.
4. Focus on items with moderate-to-high readiness or explore ways to boost readiness on lower-rated goals.

Tips for Debriefing

- Encourage honesty if they're not prepared.
- Remind them it's normal to have varying readiness for different issues.

Troubleshooting Common Challenges

- If they keep choosing low numbers, ask what would raise it by one point.
- If they inflate ratings, check if they're trying to please you or hurry therapy.

Reflection Questions

- What influences your readiness level for each goal?
- Which item stands out as a good starting place?

Real-Life Example
Caleb rated "reduce social media use" at 7/10 and "mend family ties" at 3/10. Together, they started with social media, building success before tackling family conflict.

Worksheet 7: Setting SMART Goals

Title
Setting SMART Goals

The Purpose
You transform vague wishes into concrete plans: Specific, Measurable, Achievable, Relevant, and Time-bound targets.

The Rationale

Doran (1981) introduced SMART as a framework that improves clarity and follow-through, boosting the odds of real change.

Step-by-Step Instructions

1. Pick a broad aim ("improve health").
2. Convert it into a SMART format (e.g., "I will walk for 20 minutes, three times a week, for the next month").
3. Check each letter of SMART.
4. Write it down and confirm it feels realistic.

Tips for Debriefing

- Ask if the client sees any part of the goal as ambiguous.
- Ensure they see how progress will be tracked.

Troubleshooting Common Challenges

- If it's too big, narrow it to a smaller timeframe or simpler action.
- If it's not measurable, add numeric or observable elements.

Reflection Questions

- How does having a SMART goal change your motivation?
- Which step do you find easiest to start with?

Real-Life Example

"Exercise more" became "Walk 15 minutes every Monday, Wednesday, and Friday for one month." This made the plan clear and achievable.

Worksheet 8: Ambivalence Clarification

Title

Ambivalence Clarification

The Purpose
You validate the client's mixed feelings about a particular goal, helping them see both "yes" and "no" sides clearly.

The Rationale
Miller and Rollnick (2013) say ambivalence is normal. Voicing and exploring it fosters deeper commitment once resolved.

Step-by-Step Instructions

1. Ask the client to list positives of addressing the issue and positives of not addressing it.
2. Do the same for negatives of both acting and not acting.
3. Summarise each column.
4. Discuss any real shifts in perspective.

Tips for Debriefing

- Gently highlight any contradictions.
- Encourage them to see ambivalence as part of the process.

Troubleshooting Common Challenges

- If the client feels guilty about not wanting to change, normalise that conflict.
- If the lists seem equal, look for deeper underlying priorities.

Reflection Questions

- Which side felt strongest to you?
- Did exploring both halves help you see a next step?

Real-Life Example
Victor wanted to quit smoking but feared social isolation. Listing pros and cons showed that staying healthy outweighed social concerns, motivating him to try.

Worksheet 9: Narrative Timeline

Title
Narrative Timeline

The Purpose
You plot out events or behaviours linked to a core issue over time, revealing how it developed and changed.

The Rationale
White and Epston (1990) emphasise that seeing a problem's storyline helps clients spot patterns, triggers, and progression.

Step-by-Step Instructions

1. Draw a horizontal line on paper, marking years or milestones.
2. Plot key incidents or phases related to the issue (e.g., when it started, big setbacks, small wins).
3. Note any emotional states or life events at each point.
4. Identify turning points to focus on in sessions.

Tips for Debriefing

- Observe if the timeline triggers strong memories.
- Encourage gentle self-compassion while reviewing tough events.

Troubleshooting Common Challenges

- If the client is overwhelmed by negative memories, proceed slowly, offering reassurance.
- If dates are unclear, approximate or use significant periods instead.

Reflection Questions

- Which point in your timeline stands out most?
- How might this long view help guide what you do next?

Real-Life Example
Donna created a timeline of her struggle with overeating, noticing it worsened after job stress. She saw a pattern each time work demands spiked.

Worksheet 10: Short-Term vs. Long-Term Goals

Title
Short-Term vs. Long-Term Goals

The Purpose
You separate objectives that can be met soon from those needing more time, helping the client pace their efforts wisely.

The Rationale
Locke and Latham (2002) state that distinguishing immediate targets from future aims leads to better focus and consistent motivation.

Step-by-Step Instructions

1. Divide a sheet into two columns: "Short-Term" and "Long-Term."
2. Sort the client's goals into each column.
3. Set time horizons (e.g., "Within 2 weeks," "Within 6 months").
4. Discuss how short-term steps might lay the groundwork for bigger outcomes.

Tips for Debriefing

- Validate the significance of quick wins.
- Emphasise that smaller achievements build momentum.

Troubleshooting Common Challenges

- If the client lumps everything in the near term, gently question feasibility.
- If they only list long-term ideals, brainstorm immediate steps that feed into them.

Reflection Questions

- Which short-term goal brings you the quickest sense of progress?
- How can early victories boost confidence for long-term goals?

Real-Life Example
Carlos planned to read one self-help chapter daily (short-term) while aiming to finish his degree in two years (long-term). The daily reading made him feel productive right away.

Worksheet 11: Exploring Client Expectations

Title
Exploring Client Expectations

The Purpose
You find out exactly what the client hopes therapy will look like, clarifying roles and preventing misunderstandings.

The Rationale
Swift and Greenberg (2015) demonstrate that discussing expectations aligns therapy methods with client preferences, boosting engagement.

Step-by-Step Instructions

1. Invite the client to describe what they think therapy will involve.
2. Ask about their preferred style (direct advice, reflective listening, etc.).
3. Explore what they see as signs of progress.
4. Summarise these expectations and check for any mismatch with your approach.

Tips for Debriefing

- Reassure them that sharing any concerns is welcome.
- Adjust your plan to meet reasonable preferences.

Troubleshooting Common Challenges

- If they expect instant solutions, explain how change usually takes time.
- If they have unclear expectations, provide examples of therapy processes.

Reflection Questions

- How does stating your expectations help you feel more in control?
- Which expectation do you feel is most crucial?

Real-Life Example
Katie thought therapy would be mostly advice-giving. On hearing it's more collaborative, she relaxed, feeling relieved that her viewpoint mattered.

Worksheet 12: Hierarchy of Concerns

Title
Hierarchy of Concerns

The Purpose
You ask the client to rank their problems or goals from greatest to least urgent or bothersome, clarifying where to begin.

The Rationale
Egan (2013) points out that a ranking approach highlights top issues so therapy can target the most pressing matters first.

Step-by-Step Instructions

1. Have the client list their concerns in random order.
2. Ask them to sort the list from most troubling to least.
3. Discuss why each item landed where it did.
4. Note the top 1–2 items as the immediate focus.

Tips for Debriefing

- Support the client if they feel anxious naming one concern as "biggest."
- Point out how addressing the top problem might ease smaller ones.

Troubleshooting Common Challenges

- If everything is "top priority," talk about the negative impact of scattered focus.
- If the client can't decide, weigh each item's impact on their daily life.

Reflection Questions

- Did clarifying a top concern help reduce confusion?
- Which concern do you want to tackle first?

Real-Life Example
Monica identified "panic attacks" as the biggest concern, followed by "relationship tension." She felt a sense of relief knowing where to start.

Worksheet 13: Visualising an Ideal Outcome

Title
Visualising an Ideal Outcome

The Purpose
You encourage the client to picture a successful resolution and note any feelings or benefits attached to reaching it.

The Rationale
Bandura (1997) indicates that positive visualisation can enhance belief in one's capacity to achieve a desired end result.

Step-by-Step Instructions

1. Ask the client to close their eyes and imagine the problem solved.
2. Have them describe what's different: emotions, daily routine, relationships.
3. Write down the key elements they mention.
4. Use these insights as motivation for focused work.

Tips for Debriefing

- Validate their excitement or hope.
- Discuss how reality may differ slightly but how their vision can still guide them.

Troubleshooting Common Challenges

- If the client struggles to imagine success, prompt them with questions about small improvements.
- If negative thoughts appear, acknowledge them but refocus on possibilities.

Reflection Questions

- Which parts of your vision feel most achievable right now?
- Did you feel a boost of optimism after visualising?

Real-Life Example
Sam, 22, pictured feeling calm at social events and making new friends with ease. This clear image inspired him to tackle his social anxiety step by step.

Worksheet 14: Resource Inventory

Title
Resource Inventory

The Purpose
You help the client list skills, support networks, and other assets that can assist them in pursuing their focus area.

The Rationale
Snyder et al. (2002) note that recognising available resources fosters hope and resilience, especially during challenging moments.

Step-by-Step Instructions

1. Ask the client to note personal strengths (e.g., problem-solving, empathy).
2. Add external supports: friends, family, or professionals.
3. Include practical resources like online support or local groups.
4. Discuss how each resource can be tapped to move forward.

Tips for Debriefing

- Encourage the client to see this as an empowering list.

- Check if they want to contact or activate any resource soon.

Troubleshooting Common Challenges

- If they claim no resources, gently ask about past times they overcame adversity.
- If their support system is weak, brainstorm how to build or expand it.

Reflection Questions

- Which resource seems most helpful right now?
- How can you use your personal strengths more effectively?

Real-Life Example
Jameel wrote that he's persistent, has a close sister who listens, and can access a free community workshop for job skills. This boosted his confidence in finding solutions.

Worksheet 15: Session-by-Session Plan

Title
Session-by-Session Plan

The Purpose
You outline possible milestones or topics for upcoming sessions so both you and the client have a roadmap to follow.

The Rationale
Cooper and McLeod (2011) mention that a clear session plan boosts transparency and focus, giving therapy structure without boxing it in.

Step-by-Step Instructions

1. Look at the client's top concerns or goals.
2. Sketch a rough sequence: "Session 1 – clarify goals, Session 2 – explore triggers, Session 3 – build coping tools."
3. Confirm with the client if this order feels right.
4. Adjust regularly as new insights emerge.

Tips for Debriefing

- Remind the client this plan can change.
- Let them know each session will still include flexible discussion time.

Troubleshooting Common Challenges

- If they worry about over-planning, emphasise it's just a guide.
- If they prefer spontaneity, keep the outline loose.

Reflection Questions

- Does having a roadmap reduce your worries about therapy's direction?
- Which session are you most looking forward to?

Real-Life Example
Daria accepted a 5-session outline: first addressing her childhood experiences, then step-by-step building anger management strategies.

Worksheet 16: Identify Helpful Allies

Title
Identify Helpful Allies

The Purpose
You prompt the client to find supportive people or professionals who can contribute to reaching the chosen goal.

The Rationale
Cohen (2004) found that positive social support correlates with better outcomes in managing stress and achieving personal objectives.

Step-by-Step Instructions

1. Ask the client to list friends, family, mentors, or community contacts who could help.

2. For each ally, define how they might assist (moral support, accountability check-ins, etc.).
3. Check if the client feels comfortable enlisting that person.
4. Encourage them to reach out and set up a supportive routine.

Tips for Debriefing

- Remind them that allies often appreciate being asked for help.
- Brainstorm ways to involve these allies (phone calls, in-person visits).

Troubleshooting Common Challenges

- If the client lacks social ties, discuss alternative sources (online groups, volunteer organisations).
- If they fear burdening others, gently explore that worry.

Reflection Questions

- Who has helped you in the past with similar challenges?
- How could you invite them to play a role now?

Real-Life Example
Miranda decided her sister could offer weekly check-ins about her new budgeting plan. This made the plan more real and supported.

Worksheet 17: Redefining Success

Title
Redefining Success

The Purpose
You question rigid ideas of success or failure, inviting the client to see progress as ongoing rather than all-or-nothing.

The Rationale
Brown and Ryan (2003) note that adopting flexible success definitions can lower shame and boost sustained effort during setbacks.

Step-by-Step Instructions

1. Ask how the client currently defines success for their main goal.
2. Explore alternative definitions that include partial wins (e.g., reduced frequency of a habit).
3. Write down at least three success markers, from minimal improvement to ideal results.
4. Revisit these markers regularly.

Tips for Debriefing

- If the client is perfectionistic, stress that any positive shift is worth celebrating.
- Reinforce that learning from mistakes can itself be a success.

Troubleshooting Common Challenges

- If they resist a broader view, gently ask about past times small steps led to bigger changes.
- If self-judgement persists, emphasise incremental achievements.

Reflection Questions

- How might your new definition of success encourage you to keep going?
- Which marker feels most reachable now?

Real-Life Example
Serena initially saw "total calm in all social situations" as success. After reflection, she chose "speaking up in one group meeting a week" as a success marker, reducing pressure on herself.

Worksheet 18: Accepting Multiple Foci

Title
Accepting Multiple Foci

The Purpose
You guide clients who have more than one urgent issue to merge them in an organised way rather than ignoring one.

The Rationale
Egan (2013) suggests that acknowledging multiple focal points can ease the client's tension about picking just one, while still maintaining order.

Step-by-Step Instructions

1. Invite the client to name each pressing concern (health, career, family conflict).
2. Discuss if they want to rotate attention weekly or address them in a structured sequence.
3. Write a brief plan of how each area will get time.
4. Check in each session on how the rotation or plan is working.

Tips for Debriefing

- Acknowledge that life rarely has a single issue.
- Encourage them not to feel guilt about juggling multiple goals.

Troubleshooting Common Challenges

- If they get overwhelmed, focus on simpler steps for each area.
- If one area overshadows others, remind them of the plan's balance.

Reflection Questions

- Do you feel calmer knowing we can address more than one issue over time?
- How do these different areas interact or support each other?

Real-Life Example
Carlos needed help with anxiety and career uncertainty. His therapist alternated sessions: first focusing on job strategies, next session on anxiety coping. This balanced approach lowered his stress.

Worksheet 19: When Goals Conflict

Title
When Goals Conflict

The Purpose
You help the client navigate clashing aims (e.g., wanting more free time but also wanting a demanding new job).

The Rationale
Stevens and Ricard (2016) propose that openly discussing conflicting goals prevents frustration and helps find workable compromises.

Step-by-Step Instructions

1. List each goal that seems incompatible.
2. Ask the client to outline the benefits and drawbacks of pursuing each.
3. Brainstorm creative solutions or compromises (part-time work?).
4. Choose an approach to test or a sequence to pursue.

Tips for Debriefing

- Remind them that partial satisfaction of each goal might be a good step.
- Validate any disappointment at not achieving both fully.

Troubleshooting Common Challenges

- If the client insists on having it all, point to time or energy limits.
- If tension arises, keep them grounded in practical realities.

Reflection Questions

- Which conflict is most challenging?
- Could you accept a middle path rather than an all-or-nothing result?

Real-Life Example
Toby desired daily leisure time yet wanted to start a side business. He decided to set up smaller business hours on weekends, preserving weeknights for rest.

Worksheet 20: Insightful Inquiry Questions

Title
Insightful Inquiry Questions

The Purpose
You collect open-ended prompts focused on a specific goal. This encourages the client to think more thoroughly about motives, barriers, or desired changes.

The Rationale
Hill (2010) shows that well-placed, open-ended questions prompt clients to share relevant details, leading to sharper clarity on how to move forward.

Step-by-Step Instructions

1. For each goal, draft 3–5 questions (e.g., "What made this goal important to you?").
2. During the session, ask these questions slowly, letting the client answer fully.
3. Reflect their response to confirm understanding.
4. Note any new insights that surface.

Tips for Debriefing

- Pause after each answer to allow more depth.
- If they seem stuck, rephrase or break the question down.

Troubleshooting Common Challenges

- If they reply with one-word answers, gently probe for more details.
- If they drift, refocus them on the original question.

Reflection Questions

- Which question uncovered a hidden angle to your goal?
- Did you find it helpful to explore your reasons more deeply?

Real-Life Example
Latoya's big aim was to improve communication with her partner. The prompt "What worries you most about speaking up?" led her to recall past negative experiences, clarifying her fear source.

Worksheet 21: Potential Pitfalls

Title
Potential Pitfalls

The Purpose
You encourage the client to foresee hurdles that might emerge in pursuing their main agenda, building strategies to handle them in advance.

The Rationale
Marlatt and Gordon (1985) emphasise the power of planning for setbacks, which fosters resilience and keeps progress on track.

Step-by-Step Instructions

1. Ask the client to list likely difficulties (time constraints, self-doubt).
2. For each, brainstorm at least one coping method (e.g., scheduling help, self-reassurance).
3. Write these down as a quick reference.
4. Revisit the list regularly to track if new pitfalls arise.

Tips for Debriefing

- Reinforce that lapses happen, and being prepared reduces panic.
- Remind them that spotting pitfalls early shows self-awareness.

Troubleshooting Common Challenges

- If the client can't imagine obstacles, share common ones you've seen.
- If they get discouraged, highlight how readiness can lower risks.

Reflection Questions

- Which obstacle feels most likely for you?
- How could you handle it effectively?

Real-Life Example

Adam knew he'd likely skip gym days when tired. He chose a buddy system so a friend would text him daily, cutting down no-shows.

Worksheet 22: Revisiting Motivations

Title

Revisiting Motivations

The Purpose

You circle back to why the client initially chose a certain focus, re-energising their passion and reminding them of the bigger picture.

The Rationale

Ryan and Deci (2000) found that consistent reflection on personal reasons for change fosters sustained drive, lowering the risk of giving up.

Step-by-Step Instructions

1. Pull out notes or ask, "What first motivated you about this goal?"
2. Let the client talk through any changes in their reasons.
3. If the motivation is waning, see if any new factors can reignite it.
4. Write an updated statement of motivation if needed.

Tips for Debriefing

- Notice if new life events have shifted their perspective.
- Affirm that motivations can evolve over time.

Troubleshooting Common Challenges

- If they appear bored, check if the goal is still relevant or needs reworking.
- If they rely on external pressures, guide them to find internal meaning too.

Reflection Questions

- What part of your original motivation still resonates?
- What fresh reasons might push you forward?

Real-Life Example
Chelsea wanted to lose weight because of a family wedding but later found that feeling stronger in daily tasks was her deeper incentive.

Worksheet 23: Empowerment Check

Title
Empowerment Check

The Purpose
You confirm the client truly feels ownership over the chosen focus, reducing any sense of coercion or forced direction.

The Rationale
Deci and Ryan (2008) highlight that self-determination leads to better outcomes. People flourish when they sense they're in control of their growth.

Step-by-Step Instructions

1. Ask, "Does this focus genuinely belong to you?"
2. Invite them to share any doubts or external pressures.
3. If needed, revise the plan to emphasise what they personally want.
4. Encourage them to voice opinions on pacing or method.

Tips for Debriefing

- Reinforce that therapy is their journey.
- If they mention social or family demands, see how to balance those with their own desires.

Troubleshooting Common Challenges

- If they say "I don't really want this," explore new goals or reframe the existing one.
- If they fear letting others down, empathise and see if a compromise is possible.

Reflection Questions

- Which part of this focus feels most self-chosen?
- How can you keep reminding yourself it's your decision?

Real-Life Example
Richard realised he was pushing himself to fix his marriage only because his parents urged him. Reframing the goal as "improve communication" made it feel personally meaningful.

Worksheet 24: Layered Problem Discussion

Title
Layered Problem Discussion

The Purpose
You tackle complex issues that have sub-problems, ensuring the work remains organised and not overwhelming.

The Rationale
Barkham et al. (2010) state that slicing large problems into smaller parts can reduce anxiety and make progress steps clearer.

Step-by-Step Instructions

1. Identify the overarching problem.

2. Break it into subtopics (e.g., "financial stress" might be "overspending habits," "low income," "debt management").
3. Arrange these subtopics in a logical order.
4. Plan to address each layer step by step.

Tips for Debriefing

- Validate that big problems often have multiple dimensions.
- Encourage the client not to rush all layers at once.

Troubleshooting Common Challenges

- If the client feels lost, help them define each subtopic more concretely.
- If they skip around, gently remind them of the structure.

Reflection Questions

- Which layer feels simplest to resolve?
- How do these layers interact?

Real-Life Example
Dana faced "stress at home," which turned out to include budget challenges and child-care responsibilities. Handling the budget first made child-care issues easier to handle.

Worksheet 25: Communication Style for Focusing

Title
Communication Style for Focusing

The Purpose
You practise phrasing that invites the client's preference on which goal to tackle first, fostering collaboration and respect.

The Rationale
Miller and Rollnick (2013) note that subtle language cues can shift therapy from directive to cooperative, increasing the client's sense of safety.

Step-by-Step Instructions

1. Gather your typical "focusing" questions (e.g., "Which area is most important for you right now?").
2. Replace any directive commands with these collaborative phrases.
3. During the session, use them and observe how the client responds.
4. Adjust your tone if you sense the client is unsure or hesitant.

Tips for Debriefing

- Note if the client looked more at ease deciding for themselves.
- Share how you felt using less directive language.

Troubleshooting Common Challenges

- If the client resists choosing, gently encourage them to pick the smallest or simplest item.
- If they want you to decide, remind them their voice guides therapy.

Reflection Questions

- Did these phrases help you feel more ownership?
- How did it feel being asked instead of told?

Real-Life Example

Melissa usually expected her therapist to lead. Hearing, "Which topic do you feel ready to discuss first?" led her to choose dealing with her insomnia over panic attacks initially.

Worksheet 26: Self-Reflection Prompt

Title
Self-Reflection Prompt

The Purpose

You encourage the client to keep a brief daily note or journal on their chosen focus, bringing reflections to sessions.

The Rationale

Pennebaker (1997) found that consistent journaling heightens self-awareness, aiding clients in noticing triggers or small victories.

Step-by-Step Instructions

1. Provide a short template: "Today's main thought about my goal…"
2. Ask them to write a few lines each day.
3. Request they bring these notes to the next session.
4. Discuss patterns or surprising insights they found.

Tips for Debriefing

- Encourage honesty, even if the reflection is negative or uncertain.
- Praise any consistent writing as part of the process.

Troubleshooting Common Challenges

- If they forget, remind them to set a daily reminder on their phone.
- If they resist writing, consider an audio note option.

Reflection Questions

- Did putting thoughts on paper reveal anything new?
- How did you feel revisiting your reflections in therapy?

Real-Life Example

Bella wrote a sentence each night about her mood and progress on reducing caffeine. She noticed a pattern: mood dips often triggered her to drink more coffee.

Worksheet 27: Connecting Focusing to Values

Title
Connecting Focusing to Values

The Purpose
You strengthen the link between the client's primary concern and at least one of their personal or cultural values for deeper motivation.

The Rationale
Rokeach (1973) suggests that people show stronger commitment when tasks match their core beliefs and moral principles.

Step-by-Step Instructions

1. Have the client recall their top values (kindness, honesty, tradition).
2. Ask how the focus (e.g., losing weight) supports or expresses each value.
3. Write a statement: "By doing [X], I'm living my value of [Y]."
4. Let them review and refine that statement.

Tips for Debriefing

- Highlight any emotional reaction to seeing how a goal matches values.
- Encourage them to keep this statement visible.

Troubleshooting Common Challenges

- If they see no connection, see if the focus needs tweaking or if a different value is relevant.
- If they have many values, pick the most resonant one.

Reflection Questions

- Which value connection excites or comforts you most?
- How might recalling this connection help on hard days?

Real-Life Example
Rita linked her goal of better stress management to her value of being a present mother. This emotional tie kept her motivated when learning new coping tools.

Worksheet 28: Scaling Worksheet

Title
Scaling Worksheet

The Purpose
You measure how strongly the client cares about each potential focus on a 1–10 scale, clarifying priority levels.

The Rationale
A scale approach (Murphy & Duncan, 2007) offers a simple method to gauge motivation or concern, guiding next steps.

Step-by-Step Instructions

1. List each potential target.
2. Ask the client to rate importance from 1 (very low) to 10 (very high).
3. Discuss why they chose that number.
4. Compare ratings and pick the top one or two to begin with.

Tips for Debriefing

- Explore what might raise a 6 to a 7, or keep a 9 from being a 10.
- Validate that all items matter, even if they rank lower.

Troubleshooting Common Challenges

- If everything is rated high, break them down or do a second scale for "urgency."
- If they change ratings often, check if external influences are shifting their priorities.

Reflection Questions

- Which rating surprised you the most?
- Do these numbers match how you feel day to day?

Real-Life Example

Ash gave "improving sleep" a 9 but "eating better" a 5, deciding to work on sleep first since it clearly mattered more.

Worksheet 29: Strengths-Based Agenda

Title
Strengths-Based Agenda

The Purpose
You craft an action plan focusing on the client's existing talents or successes, building optimism and self-belief.

The Rationale
Seligman (2011) emphasises leveraging strengths as a powerful route to positive change, rather than only fixing weaknesses.

Step-by-Step Instructions

1. List 2–3 strengths (e.g., determination, empathy) relevant to the main goal.
2. Brainstorm ways to apply each strength.
3. Plan steps that highlight these abilities (e.g., "Use my knack for organisation to schedule daily practice").
4. Review regularly to see how it's working.

Tips for Debriefing

- Reinforce that focusing on strengths builds confidence.
- Acknowledge any discomfort the client might feel about praising themselves.

Troubleshooting Common Challenges

- If they deny having strengths, share any you've observed.
- If they fear sounding arrogant, reassure them it's about honest self-awareness.

Reflection Questions

- Which strength do you see helping you most this week?
- How has it helped in past successes?

Real-Life Example
Jared used his "problem-solving skill" to handle small daily tasks. He found creative ways to tackle obstacles that once made him procrastinate.

Worksheet 30: Lifestyle Assessment

Title
Lifestyle Assessment

The Purpose
You explore how the targeted issue weaves into the client's daily habits and routines, spotting patterns that either support or hinder change.

The Rationale
Skinner (1953) noted that behaviour often ties to environmental cues. Understanding routine context helps fine-tune the focus.

Step-by-Step Instructions

1. Invite the client to write a typical day's schedule (wake time, meals, work, relaxation).
2. See where the focus area fits (e.g., stress peaks at midday).
3. Identify times or triggers that help or harm progress.
4. Plan adjustments or supportive routines.

Tips for Debriefing

- Notice any specific triggers (lack of sleep, missed meals).
- Affirm how small shifts can create big changes over time.

Troubleshooting Common Challenges

- If they can't see patterns, suggest journaling over a few days for more data.

- If they have an irregular schedule, adapt the approach, focusing on typical triggers.

Reflection Questions

- Did mapping your day reveal windows of opportunity or risk?
- How can you tweak your routine to support the goal?

Real-Life Example
Jean discovered that every afternoon slump led to snacking on sugary foods, derailing her plan. She decided to add a protein-filled lunch and a brisk walk instead.

Worksheet 31: Checking Commitment

Title
Checking Commitment

The Purpose
You gauge the client's level of dedication to the chosen focus, using another simple 1–10 scale but for commitment rather than importance.

The Rationale
Miller and Rollnick (2013) distinguish between importance and commitment: even if something is important, the client might not feel fully committed yet.

Step-by-Step Instructions

1. Ask, "How committed are you to working on this area?"
2. Let them pick a number from 1–10.
3. If the number is low, discuss what might raise it.
4. If it's high, plan actions matching that enthusiasm.

Tips for Debriefing

- Explore any differences between importance and commitment.
- Encourage the client to be honest if doubts remain.

Troubleshooting Common Challenges

- If they score high but show little follow-through, see if obstacles exist or if it's social desirability.
- If they hesitate, let them know it's okay to adjust the focus.

Reflection Questions

- What holds you back from a higher commitment level?
- How could you strengthen that commitment in daily life?

Real-Life Example
Becca rated her commitment to cutting down alcohol at 5, realising she needed more concrete reasons and better stress outlets to feel more devoted.

Worksheet 32: Myths vs. Reality

Title
Myths vs. Reality

The Purpose
You challenge misconceptions about therapy or about the chosen goal, ensuring the client enters the process with a balanced mindset.

The Rationale
Beck (2011) found that challenging inaccurate beliefs can reduce self-sabotage and promote realistic expectations about progress.

Step-by-Step Instructions

1. Ask the client to list any myths or assumptions about the problem or therapy (e.g., "Only weak people need therapy").
2. Offer facts or gentle challenges to these myths.
3. Replace each myth with a more accurate statement.
4. Have the client recap these new perspectives.

Tips for Debriefing

- Validate that such myths often come from culture or past experiences.
- Encourage the client to notice if they slip back into old beliefs.

Troubleshooting Common Challenges

- If they firmly hold a myth, avoid direct confrontation; ask for evidence or experiences instead.
- If new statements feel unnatural, let them refine the wording.

Reflection Questions

- Which myth did you find hardest to let go of?
- How might the new facts help you move forward?

Real-Life Example
Tina believed therapy meant being "broken." Reading studies on how therapy helps many functional people shift small habits changed her viewpoint, reducing shame.

Worksheet 33: Focus Accountability

Title
Focus Accountability

The Purpose
You create a simple tracking method where the client logs small tasks related to their main agenda. This spurs consistent effort.

The Rationale
Research by Sheldon (2014) shows that accountability measures, like weekly task logs, can double follow-through rates.

Step-by-Step Instructions

1. Define 1–3 specific weekly tasks tied to the client's focus.

2. Provide a basic chart for them to tick off each completed task.
3. Have them bring the completed chart to the next session.
4. Discuss successes and challenges, adjusting tasks as needed.

Tips for Debriefing

- Praise each completed item, however small.
- If tasks slip, help them refine or simplify them.

Troubleshooting Common Challenges

- If they forget to fill it out, have them set a reminder on their phone.
- If they feel judged, clarify that the chart is about self-awareness, not blame.

Reflection Questions

- Did seeing your progress in writing motivate you?
- How might you maintain or adjust these tasks?

Real-Life Example
Myles recorded daily steps to reduce junk food intake. Checking off "ate a healthy snack today" gave him tangible proof of progress, boosting morale.

Worksheet 34: Recalibration Exercise

Title
Recalibration Exercise

The Purpose
You periodically review the main focus with the client, confirming it still aligns with shifting life circumstances and priorities.

The Rationale
Hayes et al. (1999) suggest routine check-ins on goals helps catch changes in motivation or life context, keeping therapy relevant.

Step-by-Step Instructions

1. At scheduled intervals (monthly or after a milestone), revisit the focus.
2. Ask, "Does this still feel crucial to you? What's changed?"
3. If needed, tweak or redefine the goal.
4. Document any modifications in your notes or on a fresh worksheet.

Tips for Debriefing

- Frame recalibration as growth, not failure.
- Keep lines open for the client to share new interests or stressors.

Troubleshooting Common Challenges

- If they fear letting go of the original plan, normalise that life evolves.
- If they frequently change focus, discuss if deeper indecision is at play.

Reflection Questions

- Has something in your life shifted that affects this goal?
- Is there a simpler or more precise way to state the objective now?

Real-Life Example
Joy initially wanted to fix sleep issues. After a job change, she pivoted to stress management as her top focus. Recalibration helped her adapt therapy to her new schedule.

Worksheet 35: Underlying Beliefs

Title
Underlying Beliefs

The Purpose
You help the client uncover hidden self-talk or beliefs that keep the identified issue stuck, leading to deeper resolution.

The Rationale

Beck (2011) states that core beliefs heavily shape behaviour. Exposing them can unlock paths to healthier patterns.

Step-by-Step Instructions

1. Ask the client what thoughts come up when they think about their issue.
2. Dig deeper: "What might that say about you or the world?"
3. Note any absolute statements ("I can't succeed," "People always judge me").
4. Discuss how these beliefs affect motivation or action.

Tips for Debriefing

- Gently challenge any sweeping or harsh conclusions.
- Suggest verifying these beliefs against real-life evidence.

Troubleshooting Common Challenges

- If they resist exploring beliefs, focus on small statements first.
- If it becomes too emotional, shift to supportive affirmations and coping tools.

Reflection Questions

- Which belief surprised you once you said it aloud?
- How true does that belief still feel?

Real-Life Example

Lucy discovered she believed, "I'm not worthy of good things," blocking her from applying for better jobs. Recognising it helped her question it and try new steps.

Worksheet 36: Flexible Goal Setting

Title

Flexible Goal Setting

The Purpose
You highlight that targets can be modified when life changes or if the original plan proves unworkable, preventing feelings of defeat.

The Rationale
Norcross et al. (2011) suggest that adapting goals is essential. Sticking rigidly to a failing plan can halt progress and crush morale.

Step-by-Step Instructions

1. Ask the client to review their current goals.
2. Discuss any shifts in time, resources, or personal interest.
3. Amend the goal as needed (lowering or raising difficulty, changing timelines).
4. Ensure the new version still feels meaningful.

Tips for Debriefing

- Use examples of real people who adapted goals successfully.
- Reassure them that changing a plan is not quitting.

Troubleshooting Common Challenges

- If they resist changing a plan, validate loyalty but emphasise results.
- If they keep altering goals without action, explore what's blocking follow-through.

Reflection Questions

- What has changed that makes the original goal less fitting now?
- How does the new version energise or excite you?

Real-Life Example
Ava's aim to read a book weekly became unrealistic after her workload jumped. Adjusting it to "finish two books a month" helped her stay on track.

Worksheet 37: Strategic Decision Tree

Title
Strategic Decision Tree

The Purpose
You map out possible choices, outcomes, and next steps, letting the client see how each path could unfold.

The Rationale
Hammond et al. (1999) recommend decision trees to organise complex decisions, promoting clarity about potential results.

Step-by-Step Instructions

1. Write a key decision at the trunk (e.g., "Switch jobs or stay").
2. Branch out two or more paths.
3. Under each path, list possible outcomes or barriers.
4. Explore how the client feels about each scenario.

Tips for Debriefing

- Guide them to notice emotional responses to each path.
- Emphasise that no path is perfect, but each might hold benefits.

Troubleshooting Common Challenges

- If the client gets overwhelmed, start with just two main branches.
- If they want a guaranteed outcome, discuss realistic unpredictability.

Reflection Questions

- Which branch looks most appealing?
- What does your gut say about the likely best route?

Real-Life Example
Jake considered "quit job vs. stay." The "quit job" branch included short-term financial strain but potential happiness in a new field. Visualising this helped him weigh pros and cons calmly.

Worksheet 38: Time Allocation Chart

Title
Time Allocation Chart

The Purpose
You ask the client to log weekly activities, spotting if their actual schedule matches the chosen focus or if adjustments are needed.

The Rationale
Claessens et al. (2007) show that tracking time use can highlight gaps or over-commitments, enabling more effective planning.

Step-by-Step Instructions

1. Provide a simple grid with days and hours.
2. Have the client fill in how they spend each block of time.
3. Compare usage to their main priority (e.g., if they want more exercise but never schedule it).
4. Brainstorm changes in the schedule to align it with the focus.

Tips for Debriefing

- Acknowledge that seeing the chart can be eye-opening.
- Suggest micro-changes (e.g., 15-minute slots) if they can't find big chunks of free time.

Troubleshooting Common Challenges

- If they skip logging, encourage short daily updates to avoid forgetting.
- If they're overwhelmed by many responsibilities, see if certain tasks can be delegated or reduced.

Reflection Questions

- What surprised you about how you currently spend your time?
- Which task can you modify to free space for your goal?

Real-Life Example

Jack aimed to practise guitar daily but found he spent hours scrolling social media. He replaced 30 minutes of that habit with guitar practice, making real progress.

Worksheet 39: Celebrating Milestones

Title
Celebrating Milestones

The Purpose
You encourage the client to recognise each achievement tied to the focus, reinforcing motivation and positive feelings.

The Rationale
Seligman (2011) suggests that celebrating even small wins builds momentum and increases resilience against setbacks.

Step-by-Step Instructions

1. Define milestone points (e.g., finishing a week of a new routine).
2. Decide a simple reward or acknowledgment (relaxing activity, journaling about the success).
3. Encourage them to share with a supportive person if comfortable.
4. Log each milestone to see accumulating success.

Tips for Debriefing

- Ask the client how celebrating made them feel.
- Reinforce that recognition is not bragging but honouring progress.

Troubleshooting Common Challenges

- If they downplay successes, remind them that progress is progress, no matter how small.
- If they rely only on external praise, explore ways to develop internal validation too.

Reflection Questions

- Which accomplishment do you feel proudest about so far?
- What kind of celebration feels most meaningful to you?

Real-Life Example

Freya celebrated each week of consistent meal planning by taking a relaxing bath on Sunday evening. This small ritual helped her feel proud and motivated.

Worksheet 40: Focus Summary Sheet

Title

Focus Summary Sheet

The Purpose

You consolidate everything learned: the main target, reasons for choosing it, resources, strengths, obstacles, and next steps.

The Rationale

Cooper and McLeod (2011) highlight the value of a summary that brings coherence. The client sees a clear snapshot of the work ahead.

Step-by-Step Instructions

1. At the end of this focusing phase, create one page that includes:
   - The main issue.
   - The client's motivation.
   - Strengths and resources.
   - Potential pitfalls.
   - Action items or goals.
2. Review it together, ensuring accuracy.
3. Keep a copy to reference in upcoming sessions.

Tips for Debriefing

- Ask how seeing all details in one place feels.

- Encourage them to treat it like a roadmap, revisiting as needed.

Troubleshooting Common Challenges

- If it's overwhelming, emphasise it's a guide, not a rigid contract.
- If parts seem outdated, agree to revise regularly.

Reflection Questions

- Which part of the summary sheet motivates you the most?
- How might you use this sheet to stay focused between sessions?

Real-Life Example
Mia's summary sheet listed "reduce panic attacks" as her main issue, with motivations ("be more present with family"), resources (close friend for check-ins), and steps (weekly therapy tasks). She felt organised and hopeful.

With these 40 worksheets, you and your client can map out a path that aligns with their core desires and practical realities. By clarifying goals, identifying resources, and staying flexible, you'll create a well-structured framework for meaningful progress.

Evoking Change Talk

These exercises aim to draw out the client's own arguments for making changes. By highlighting desire, ability, reasons, and need (DARN), you strengthen intrinsic motivation. This category promotes self-driven solutions, harnessing the client's inner resolve rather than imposing external directives.

Worksheet 1: Desire, Ability, Reasons, and Need

Title
Desire, Ability, Reasons, and Need

The Purpose
You guide your client to identify these four elements—Desire, Ability, Reasons, Need—behind their wish to make a change.

The Rationale
Miller and Rollnick (2013) argue that clarifying each element helps clients voice solid motivations. By pinpointing how much they *want* change, *can* achieve it, *why* it matters, and *how urgent* it is, they strengthen their commitment.

Step-by-Step Instructions

1. Draw four columns labeled Desire, Ability, Reasons, Need.
2. Encourage your client to note statements matching each category.
3. Ask how each statement feels in terms of sincerity.
4. Highlight the category that has the most energy for them.

Tips for Debriefing

- Reinforce that all four components play a role.
- Compare Desire versus Need to uncover urgency.

Troubleshooting Common Challenges

- If the client struggles with one category, prompt gentle questions like, "Why else might you want this?"
- If answers are vague, help them phrase statements more clearly.

Reflection Questions

- Which category came most naturally to you?
- Do you see one category sparking more motivation?

Real life application

Linda realised she strongly *wanted* more energy (Desire), had decent time management skills (Ability), craved better health outcomes (Reasons), and felt her aches wouldn't improve unless she acted (Need). Seeing it all laid out deepened her resolve to start a fitness routine.

Worksheet 2: Visualization of a Changed Future

Title
Visualization of a Changed Future

The Purpose
You help your client imagine life post-change, tapping into uplifting feelings that can fuel progress.

The Rationale
Bandura (1997) found that mentally rehearsing success boosts confidence. By visualising their future state, clients see the emotional payoffs that keep them determined.

Step-by-Step Instructions

1. Ask your client to close their eyes or write about a day in their changed life.
2. Encourage detail: setting, emotions, positive outcomes.
3. Have them note how they feel describing this vision.
4. Discuss ways to keep this picture in mind daily.

Tips for Debriefing

- Reinforce any hopeful emotions.
- Address any anxieties that arise, reminding them it's a safe mental exercise.

Troubleshooting Common Challenges

- If they can't picture success, start with small improvements.
- If negative images appear, gently refocus on constructive possibilities.

Reflection Questions

- What part of your imagined future excites you most?
- How can you use this vision to stay motivated?

Real life application
Elliot pictured himself feeling energised at work, free from constant fatigue. He saw himself smiling more, focusing better, and enjoying time with his family. Recalling this vision daily reminded him why small lifestyle changes mattered.

Worksheet 3: Scaling Importance

Title
Scaling Importance

The Purpose
You measure how crucial the client sees the change, prompting reflection on ways to raise that importance score.

The Rationale
Rollnick and Allison (2004) emphasise that assigning a numeric value can clarify priorities. Clients then consider what could nudge that rating higher.

Step-by-Step Instructions

1. Ask, "On a scale of 1–10, how important is making this change?"
2. Invite them to explain their number.
3. Inquire, "What might move it up by one point?"
4. Brainstorm small tweaks or extra support to boost the rating.

Tips for Debriefing

- Confirm the client owns their final score.
- Notice language shifts when they see ways to increase motivation.

Troubleshooting Common Challenges

- If the score is very low, explore the cost of not changing.
- If it's high but no action follows, look for hidden barriers.

Reflection Questions

- Why did you pick that number instead of something lower?
- Which next step could raise your score slightly?

Real life application
Mia rated change importance at 6. Realising an extra 2 points could come from scheduling supportive chats with her friend, she bumped her plan to a 7, feeling more serious about quitting smoking.

Worksheet 4: Confidence Boost

Title
Confidence Boost

The Purpose
You measure the client's self-belief in making the change. This reveals areas needing reinforcement or strategy.

The Rationale
Bandura (1997) stresses self-efficacy as central to change. If clients trust their capability, they're more likely to persevere.

Step-by-Step Instructions

1. Ask, "On a scale of 1–10, how confident are you in making this change?"
2. Explore reasons for that rating.
3. Prompt, "What might raise it by one point?"
4. Discuss strategies or resources that could boost confidence.

Tips for Debriefing

- Remind them it's normal to start with a modest score.

- Identify past successes to show they can achieve more than they think.

Troubleshooting Common Challenges

- If they overestimate, suggest they consider small obstacles to keep it realistic.
- If they underrate, highlight strengths you observe.

Reflection Questions

- How does noticing your confidence level affect your next move?
- Which resource would help you feel more certain?

Real life application
Ron rated himself at 4 for tackling social anxiety. Remembering a time he succeeded in giving a speech, he realised he could push that to 5 by practising deep breathing, then tried attending a small group event.

Worksheet 5: Change Talk Brainstorm

Title
Change Talk Brainstorm

The Purpose
You prompt clients to list any reason for changing, uncovering small sparks that can ignite stronger motivation.

The Rationale
Miller and Rollnick (2013) show that gathering "change talk" phrases helps clients hear their own push for action, making it harder to ignore.

Step-by-Step Instructions

1. Set a timer for three minutes.
2. Ask clients to write every reason they can think of for changing.
3. Encourage them not to filter or judge their ideas.
4. Review the list, highlighting the strongest or most heartfelt reasons.

Tips for Debriefing

- Applaud each reason, even small ones.
- Ask which reason they feel ready to commit to first.

Troubleshooting Common Challenges

- If they stall, mention areas like health, finances, relationships for inspiration.
- If they only list negatives, ask for at least one potential positive.

Reflection Questions

- Which reasons resonate with you most right now?
- How might you use this list during moments of doubt?

Real life application

Tanya wrote many reasons to cut back on sugar: avoiding diabetes, feeling more energetic, improving skin. Focusing on "feeling lighter daily" energised her to pick fruit instead of chocolate bars.

Worksheet 6: Exploring Past Successes

Title
Exploring Past Successes

The Purpose
You help the client remember a time they overcame a difficulty, showing them strategies or strengths they can apply now.

The Rationale
Bandura (1997) argues that recalling triumphs boosts a client's perception of their capabilities, fostering renewed confidence.

Step-by-Step Instructions

1. Ask about a challenge they conquered before.

2. Identify what tactics or supports worked.
3. Compare that situation to the current goal, spotting parallels.
4. Plan to reuse or adapt those winning tactics.

Tips for Debriefing

- Reinforce the idea that success wasn't luck but effort and resourcefulness.
- Encourage them to see how those skills can be replicated.

Troubleshooting Common Challenges

- If they can't recall big triumphs, even small wins count.
- If they discount their achievements, gently remind them of their efforts.

Reflection Questions

- Which of your strengths stood out in that past success?
- How can it guide you now?

Real life application
Sarah overcame a fear of public speaking by practising before friends. Now, wanting to socialise more, she used the same incremental approach: talking to one or two new people each week, building confidence step by step.

Worksheet 7: Future Letter

Title
Future Letter

The Purpose
You encourage the client to imagine life after successful change, writing a short note from future self to present self, boosting hope.

The Rationale
Sheldon and Lyubomirsky (2006) show that envisioning a positive future fosters determination. This exercise turns potential dreams into encouraging words.

Step-by-Step Instructions

1. Ask the client to envision themselves months or a year from now, having made the change.
2. Write a brief letter from that perspective: "Dear me, I'm proud you stuck with it…"
3. Reflect on how it feels to read encouraging words from "future them."
4. Suggest keeping the letter as a reminder.

Tips for Debriefing

- Emphasise creativity—there's no right or wrong.
- Encourage them to read it when motivation dips.

Troubleshooting Common Challenges

- If they find it silly, frame it as a fun imaginative exercise.
- If negative future visions appear, steer them toward balanced or hopeful possibilities.

Reflection Questions

- Which part of your letter felt most uplifting?
- How might your future self want you to handle obstacles now?

Real life application

Kevin wrote, "I'm glad you believed in yourself despite setbacks. I feel healthier and prouder each day." Reading this boosted his resolve to attend therapy sessions regularly.

Worksheet 8: Reasons and Need Collage

Title
Reasons and Need Collage

The Purpose
You let visually oriented clients create a collage capturing why this change matters, anchoring them in powerful emotional images.

The Rationale
Edwards (2014) notes that art-based methods can access deeper motivations. A collage offers a strong symbolic reminder of their aspirations.

Step-by-Step Instructions

1. Provide old magazines, scissors, glue, or digital collage tools.
2. Have them pick images or words that represent their reasons and sense of urgency.
3. Assemble the collage in a way that feels meaningful.
4. Ask them to describe the final product's main messages.

Tips for Debriefing

- Explore any surprising pictures or themes.
- Suggest displaying it at home to reinforce daily motivation.

Troubleshooting Common Challenges

- If materials are limited, have them sketch or write brief keywords.
- If they feel shy, reassure them it's personal expression, not about art skills.

Reflection Questions

- Which part of your collage speaks loudest to you?
- How will you remember these reasons day to day?

Real life application
Jess created a poster with beach scenery (health), family photos (being active for loved ones), and keywords like "energy" and "freedom." Glancing at it each morning reminded her why exercise mattered so much.

Worksheet 9: Evoking from Ambivalence

Title
Evoking from Ambivalence

The Purpose
You help clients explore both the upsides and downsides of not changing versus making a change, leading them to highlight potential benefits.

The Rationale
Miller and Rollnick (2013) stress that exploring ambivalence is normal. When clients weigh each side, they often find fresh motivation.

Step-by-Step Instructions

1. Fold a sheet in half.
2. On the left, list pros and cons of staying the same.
3. On the right, list pros and cons of changing.
4. Discuss any realisation from seeing them side by side.

Tips for Debriefing

- Encourage honesty, even if it feels contradictory.
- Ask which side the client leans toward after reflection.

Troubleshooting Common Challenges

- If the pros of staying stuck dominate, revisit deeper values or future vision.
- If the client remains torn, normalise that as part of the process.

Reflection Questions

- Which con is hardest to ignore?
- How does seeing benefits of change shift your mindset?

Real life application
Ben saw that not quitting sugary drinks let him have quick pleasure but risked health

issues. Realising the long-term drawbacks outweighed short-term comfort pushed him to reduce his daily intake.

Worksheet 10: Amplifying Change Statements

Title
Amplifying Change Statements

The Purpose
You echo and enhance small hints of readiness or ability to change, boosting the client's confidence.

The Rationale
Miller and Rollnick (2013) demonstrate that focusing on positive language can expand a client's commitment to act.

Step-by-Step Instructions

1. Listen for phrases like "Maybe I could…"
2. Repeat them with emphasis: "It sounds like you really *could* do that."
3. Ask the client how it feels to hear that re-stated strongly.
4. Note any momentum or further ideas that arise.

Tips for Debriefing

- Don't force positivity; simply highlight existing sparks.
- Reinforce each step from "I might" to "I will."

Troubleshooting Common Challenges

- If they backtrack, reflect their hesitancy too.
- If they seem uneasy, keep your tone gentle and supportive.

Reflection Questions

- Did hearing your own words amplified change your perspective?

- Which statement feels stronger now?

Real life application
Shaina offhandedly said, "I guess I'd try therapy if it might help." The therapist repeated, "So you're open to giving therapy a genuine shot?" That small shift made her more likely to schedule a session.

Worksheet 11: Sorting Motivations

Title
Sorting Motivations

The Purpose
You list possible motivations—family, health, finances—and ask your client to rank them. This reveals their top reasons for change.

The Rationale
Deci and Ryan (2008) found that personal relevance elevates drive. Identifying the strongest motivator helps anchor future plans.

Step-by-Step Instructions

1. Write a set of motivations on index cards or a sheet.
2. Have the client arrange them from most to least important.
3. Discuss why the top ones rank highest.
4. Connect the leading motivators to small action steps.

Tips for Debriefing

- Explore how the top motivator can serve as daily inspiration.
- Affirm that lower-ranked ones can still matter later.

Troubleshooting Common Challenges

- If they can't decide, ask open-ended questions about their daily life.
- If they rank everything equally, propose focusing on just two for now.

Reflection Questions

- How does seeing your top motivators affect your feelings about change?
- Which area do you want to act on first?

Real life application
Maria discovered "being an example for my daughter" outweighed other reasons to lose weight. Keeping that top priority in mind helped her skip late-night snacks.

Worksheet 12: Three Good Things

Title
Three Good Things

The Purpose
You invite clients to name three potential positives from making the change, focusing on the bright side to inspire action.

The Rationale
Seligman et al. (2005) show that dwelling on positives fosters hope, which can overcome inertia or worry.

Step-by-Step Instructions

1. Ask, "What three good things might happen if you commit to this goal?"
2. Write each benefit in clear, specific wording.
3. Reflect how these outcomes align with personal values.
4. Encourage keeping the list visible or reading it before tricky moments.

Tips for Debriefing

- Validate each benefit, large or small.
- Help them see how each good thing is within reach if they stay consistent.

Troubleshooting Common Challenges

- If they only see one, gently brainstorm smaller but meaningful gains.
- If they're stuck, prompt them about relationships, health, or finances.

Reflection Questions

- Which benefit stands out most?
- How might focusing on these positives reshape your efforts?

Real life application
Renee named "less stress, feeling happier, fewer arguments at home" as her three good things from reducing screen time. Glancing at this list each day reminded her to unplug when tempted.

Worksheet 13: Potential Consequences of Inaction

Title
Potential Consequences of Inaction

The Purpose
You encourage reflection on what happens if nothing changes, clarifying the costs of maintaining the status quo.

The Rationale
Miller and Rollnick (2013) emphasise exploring inaction's risks can prompt a client to see how vital forward steps are.

Step-by-Step Instructions

1. Ask, "What might happen if you continue as is for another year?"
2. Let them list possible outcomes—physical, emotional, social.
3. Compare these to the desired scenario.
4. Check if acknowledging these downsides raises their motivation.

Tips for Debriefing

- Approach gently, as the realisation can be upsetting.

- Reassure them it's normal to fear looking ahead.

Troubleshooting Common Challenges

- If the client becomes anxious, guide them to see this as a wake-up call, not a condemnation.
- If they downplay concerns, ask about past experiences or patterns.

Reflection Questions

- Which possible consequence worries you most?
- How does picturing it affect your readiness to act?

Real life application

Kurt recognised that ignoring his diet might lead to worsening health. The thought of feeling constantly exhausted pushed him to seek nutritional advice.

Worksheet 14: Role Model Reflection

Title

Role Model Reflection

The Purpose

You help your client identify someone who accomplished a similar change, then glean motivation and tactics from that example.

The Rationale

Lockwood and Kunda (1997) suggest that seeing others succeed encourages self-belief and provides practical lessons.

Step-by-Step Instructions

1. Ask, "Who do you know—real or famous—who overcame something like this?"
2. List qualities or steps they took.
3. Discuss how those strategies could be adapted.

4. Have the client note which lessons resonate most.

Tips for Debriefing

- Reinforce uniqueness: they don't have to mimic the role model exactly.
- Praise the idea of learning from someone else's journey.

Troubleshooting Common Challenges

- If they can't think of anyone, explore online success stories or supportive groups.
- If they feel "not good enough," gently reframe that they can adopt small steps.

Reflection Questions

- Which quality of your role model do you admire most?
- How can you incorporate that trait into your approach?

Real life application
Drew thought of a friend who beat depression through steady therapy and exercise. Inspired, he decided to combine counselling with regular walks to replicate a similar path.

Worksheet 15: Evoking Autonomy

Title
Evoking Autonomy

The Purpose
You remind the client they are free to choose or refuse each step, reinforcing a sense of ownership.

The Rationale
Deci and Ryan (2008) show that people thrive when they feel they're in control. Honouring their autonomy nurtures genuine engagement.

Step-by-Step Instructions

1. Emphasise: "You get to decide if, how, and when you act."
2. Explore whether this freedom sparks relief or anxiety.
3. Suggest small steps if they request direction but never impose.
4. Reflect their words back, showing respect for their freedom to pivot.

Tips for Debriefing

- Watch for a shift in posture or tone when they realise they're in charge.
- Validate any mixed feelings about responsibility.

Troubleshooting Common Challenges

- If they want direct orders, gently reaffirm that real change is self-chosen.
- If they feel pressured, reassure them they can slow down or adjust the goal.

Reflection Questions

- How does recognising your power to choose alter your motivation?
- Which decision feels important to make now?

Real life application
Leila felt everyone pushed her to quit her job. Hearing "It's your decision entirely" relieved her. She decided to put in flexible job applications, feeling more in command of her life.

Worksheet 16: Change Language Rating

Title
Change Language Rating

The Purpose
You list or record the client's statements about change, then label them as weak, moderate, or strong to gauge their readiness.

The Rationale

Miller and Rollnick (2013) argue that noting the intensity of change talk can shape how you respond, fostering stronger resolve.

Step-by-Step Instructions

1. During or after the session, note key phrases: "I might…," "I will…," "I hate this habit."
2. Classify them as weak ("maybe"), moderate ("I'd like to"), or strong ("I'm done waiting").
3. Discuss how to elevate weak statements to more certain language.
4. Encourage them to adopt stronger phrasing in daily life.

Tips for Debriefing

- Highlight growth if they move from "maybe" to "I will."
- Keep the tone supportive, not judgmental.

Troubleshooting Common Challenges

- If they feel judged, explain you're simply capturing how firmly they speak about change.
- If they remain mostly in weak talk, explore deeper reasons for hesitancy.

Reflection Questions

- Which statements already sound strong?
- How can you strengthen weaker ones?

Real life application

Naomi heard herself say, "I might quit smoking someday." After rating it weak, she shifted to, "I want to quit in the next month," marking a more serious commitment.

Worksheet 17: Identifying Inconsistent Behaviours

Title
Identifying Inconsistent Behaviours

The Purpose
You help the client recognise actions that clash with their stated priorities, prompting a desire to resolve these mismatches.

The Rationale
Festinger (1957) posits that seeing one's own contradictions often inspires realignment to reduce discomfort.

Step-by-Step Instructions

1. Ask the client to name key values or objectives.
2. List behaviours from the past week.
3. Place a check next to those supporting values, and note any contradictions.
4. Reflect on how they feel seeing mismatched patterns.

Tips for Debriefing

- Focus on self-awareness rather than blame.
- Emphasise small adjustments can restore alignment.

Troubleshooting Common Challenges

- If they become defensive, reassure them it's common to slip from ideals.
- If the mismatch is huge, break it into simpler fixes.

Reflection Questions

- How did spotting these mismatches influence your motivation?
- Which small behaviour can you modify right away?

Real life application
Ollie valued honesty but regularly made excuses at work. Seeing the conflict made him decide to apologise for a recent lie and commit to openness, reducing internal tension.

Worksheet 18: Skill Confidence Building

Title
Skill Confidence Building

The Purpose
You target specific abilities needed for change, rating confidence in each so the client can focus on areas needing practice or support.

The Rationale
Bandura (1997) emphasises that improving self-efficacy in specific skills boosts overall progress.

Step-by-Step Instructions

1. List the top 3–5 skills crucial for their goal (e.g., meal planning, time scheduling).
2. Rate confidence from 1–10 for each.
3. Identify resources or steps to raise lower scores.
4. Track improvement over time.

Tips for Debriefing

- Praise existing strengths.
- Brainstorm ways to develop each skill (tutorials, mentor, practice tasks).

Troubleshooting Common Challenges

- If scores are all low, pick one easy skill to boost first.
- If they can't identify needed skills, break the goal into daily tasks.

Reflection Questions

- Which skill rating surprises you?
- How can we boost your weakest skill a bit?

Real life application
Miguel aimed to handle finances better. He rated "budgeting knowledge" at 3,

"tracking expenses" at 5, and "saving discipline" at 2. He read articles on budgeting, raised his scores gradually, and felt more empowered.

Worksheet 19: Encountering Obstacles

Title
Encountering Obstacles

The Purpose
You encourage the client to anticipate barriers to their goal and plan solutions, reducing surprises and building resilience.

The Rationale
Marlatt and Gordon (1985) note that anticipating obstacles makes relapse or setbacks less likely. Preparedness boosts confidence.

Step-by-Step Instructions

1. Ask the client to brainstorm possible hurdles.
2. For each, discuss an action or resource to cope.
3. Record the plan: "If [Obstacle], then I will [Solution]."
4. Check in regularly to update strategies.

Tips for Debriefing

- Remind them that obstacles are normal, not evidence they can't succeed.
- Revisit after each small roadblock to refine tactics.

Troubleshooting Common Challenges

- If they're stumped, share common pitfalls others face.
- If too many obstacles appear, group them or address the most urgent first.

Reflection Questions

- Which obstacle do you worry about most?

- How does having a plan ease your concerns?

Real life application
Hannah feared eating junk food when stressed. She decided that if a rough day hits, she'd call her supportive friend or keep healthy snacks at home, so temptation was lower.

Worksheet 20: Motivation Timelines

Title
Motivation Timelines

The Purpose
You chart the client's motivation highs and lows over time, seeing patterns that may guide better planning.

The Rationale
Prochaska and DiClemente (1983) show that readiness to change evolves. Mapping its fluctuations can uncover triggers or supportive factors.

Step-by-Step Instructions

1. Draw a horizontal line (timeline).
2. Mark periods (weeks, months) along it.
3. Plot points for motivation levels (1–10) over each segment.
4. Note any events correlated with rises or dips in motivation.

Tips for Debriefing

- Encourage the client to reflect on what boosted or hurt motivation at each point.
- Suggest repeating the timeline in future to spot changes.

Troubleshooting Common Challenges

- If details are foggy, approximate.

- If the pattern isn't clear, look for recurring themes like stress or support presence.

Reflection Questions

- What boosted your motivation during the highest points?
- How can we replicate those conditions or influences now?

Real life application
Dan graphed his months of working out. He saw motivation peaked when he had a gym buddy. Realising that, he teamed up with a friend again to recapture that boost.

Worksheet 21: Positive Self-Talk

Title
Positive Self-Talk

The Purpose
You help clients replace harsh inner language with supportive phrases, keeping morale high during challenging times.

The Rationale
Meichenbaum (1977) found that shifting negative self-statements to encouraging ones can bolster resilience and goal achievement.

Step-by-Step Instructions

1. Ask the client what self-criticism they often repeat.
2. Collaboratively craft a kinder, realistic phrase (e.g., "I learn from mistakes and keep trying").
3. Encourage practising this phrase daily.
4. Check how it influences their mood or readiness to act.

Tips for Debriefing

- Remind them it's normal to slip into old habits sometimes.

- Praise any small shift in internal dialogue.

Troubleshooting Common Challenges

- If they feel silly, remind them that self-talk is powerful, even if it feels odd initially.
- If their negative talk is severe, consider deeper cognitive restructuring.

Reflection Questions

- Which new phrase resonates most with you?
- How can you remind yourself to use it regularly?

Real life application
Adam caught himself saying, "I always fail." Changing it to, "I learn from setbacks and keep moving," helped him continue job searches even after rejections.

Worksheet 22: Accountability Partner

Title
Accountability Partner

The Purpose
You guide your client to find a supportive individual who can encourage, check in, or track their progress, increasing follow-through.

The Rationale
Baumeister and Leary (1995) show that social connectedness promotes commitment. Having someone to answer to often raises effort.

Step-by-Step Instructions

1. Brainstorm people they trust or admire.
2. Decide how often they'd like to check in—daily, weekly.
3. Clarify the partner's role (reminders, shared goals).
4. Encourage them to discuss boundaries or style that fits both parties.

Tips for Debriefing

- Emphasise mutual respect if they pick a close friend.
- Suggest ways to thank or reciprocate that support.

Troubleshooting Common Challenges

- If no friend or family is suitable, try online groups or community forums.
- If friction arises with the chosen partner, reevaluate frequency or type of support.

Reflection Questions

- Who in your life can compassionately hold you accountable?
- How will you communicate your needs to them?

Real life application
Ruby asked her cousin to text her each morning to confirm she was up for a jog. This daily nudge prevented her from hitting snooze out of habit.

Worksheet 23: Change Mantra

Title
Change Mantra

The Purpose
You assist the client in creating a short, powerful phrase that embodies their motivation, repeating it to reinforce determination.

The Rationale
Seligman (2011) suggests concise affirmations can anchor a person's drive, guiding them through obstacles with a clear reminder of their purpose.

Step-by-Step Instructions

1. Ask the client to distil their reason for change into a few words, like "Stronger every day."
2. Ensure it feels authentic, not forced.
3. Suggest they say it silently or aloud each morning.
4. Check in if it remains relevant or needs revision over time.

Tips for Debriefing

- Encourage them to write it somewhere visible.
- Reflect how reciting it might shift their mindset in stress moments.

Troubleshooting Common Challenges

- If they can't find the right words, revisit prior worksheets for key phrases.
- If they view mantras as silly, emphasise it's just a tool for focus.

Reflection Questions

- Does saying this phrase spark an emotional response?
- How might you use it when tempted to quit?

Real life application
Sam's mantra, "Calm and focused," echoed in his mind whenever he felt anxious about studying. This simple reminder helped him stay on track instead of panicking.

Worksheet 24: Exploring Emotional Triggers

Title
Exploring Emotional Triggers

The Purpose
You invite the client to notice which feelings—anger, fear, joy—propel them to consider change, highlighting emotional catalysts.

The Rationale

Kassianos et al. (2016) note that emotions often drive decisions. Recognising these triggers can sharpen insight into motivation.

Step-by-Step Instructions

1. Ask, "Which emotions do you feel when you think about changing (or not changing)?"
2. Note each emotion's impact.
3. Discuss ways to use beneficial emotions or handle challenging ones.
4. Encourage quick logs of emotional states around big decisions.

Tips for Debriefing

- Normalise strong emotions.
- Emphasise that fear or frustration can become fuel for action if managed well.

Troubleshooting Common Challenges

- If they aren't used to naming feelings, offer prompts like anger, guilt, hope.
- If intense emotions surface, proceed gently.

Reflection Questions

- Which emotion pushes you forward most strongly?
- How can you channel it constructively?

Real life application

Mike felt anger at losing job opportunities. Realising that anger was a sign he valued respect and stability, he channelled it into practising interview skills daily.

Worksheet 25: When a Setback Occurs

Title

When a Setback Occurs

The Purpose
You help the client devise a plan for handling inevitable setbacks, framing them as learning experiences instead of final failures.

The Rationale
Marlatt and Gordon (1985) highlight relapse prevention strategies, showing that planning for slips reduces panic and fosters resilience.

Step-by-Step Instructions

1. Brainstorm a plausible slip-up scenario.
2. Outline how they'll pause, reflect, and regroup.
3. Include who they might contact for support.
4. Encourage viewing a setback as a temporary challenge to overcome.

Tips for Debriefing

- Reinforce that one slip doesn't undo all progress.
- Suggest they re-check their motivation or use a coping skill promptly.

Troubleshooting Common Challenges

- If they see any lapse as total failure, gently remind them of partial successes.
- If they become discouraged, revisit their successes or mantra.

Reflection Questions

- How can you keep perspective if things go wrong?
- Who could offer you a kind word or boost then?

Real life application
Laura expected a possible relapse into overeating when stressed. She prepped a short list of calming activities and texted a close friend whenever she felt tempted, bouncing back faster each time.

Worksheet 26: Celebration Visualization

Title
Celebration Visualization

The Purpose
You ask the client to picture a future moment of successfully meeting their goal, tapping into emotions of pride and relief to boost drive.

The Rationale
Emmons and McCullough (2003) found that savouring imagined celebrations can energise ongoing efforts, providing a taste of the future reward.

Step-by-Step Instructions

1. Guide them to visualise the day they accomplish the goal—who's present, what's said, how they feel.
2. Ask them to describe each detail.
3. Reflect the excitement or satisfaction you hear.
4. Suggest using this mental image when feeling unmotivated.

Tips for Debriefing

- Encourage them to savour positive emotions, anchoring them to keep going.
- Check for any hidden doubts overshadowing the joy.

Troubleshooting Common Challenges

- If they struggle to celebrate themselves, propose a small milestone event.
- If they only foresee negativity, gently refocus on potential joys.

Reflection Questions

- What stands out most in your celebration scene?
- How might you keep that vision alive in daily life?

Real life application
Karen pictured a barbecue where she confidently wore clothes that once didn't fit, and her friends congratulated her. That vivid image reminded her to persist with healthier habits.

Worksheet 27: Translating Change Talk into Goals

Title
Translating Change Talk into Goals

The Purpose
You convert expressions of desire or ability ("I want to…," "I could…") into specific, achievable steps, boosting momentum.

The Rationale
Miller and Rollnick (2013) underscore the importance of moving from vague talk to concrete plans. Action steps make intentions real.

Step-by-Step Instructions

1. Listen for "I should…" or "I want to…" statements.
2. Help them clarify: "That sounds great. How will you do it?"
3. Encourage a simple, time-bound goal.
4. Write it down and revisit progress next time.

Tips for Debriefing

- Keep a supportive tone.
- Emphasise small steps if the client seems overwhelmed.

Troubleshooting Common Challenges

- If they hesitate, break the goal into a micro-step.
- If they frequently talk but never plan, ask what blocks them from commitment.

Reflection Questions

- Which statement do you want to convert into a goal today?
- What's your timeline for acting on it?

Real life application
Tom said, "I really want to cut back on late-night gaming." The therapist replied, "Let's map that. Are you ready to limit screen time after 9 p.m.?" That became his first mini-goal.

Worksheet 28: Daily Motivation Tracker

Title
Daily Motivation Tracker

The Purpose
You encourage the client to rate motivation each day, spotting patterns and intervening when low motivation shows up.

The Rationale
Sheldon (2014) notes that regular self-monitoring helps clients see fluctuations and practice strategies to sustain drive.

Step-by-Step Instructions

1. Give them a simple grid—days of the week in one column, a 1–10 motivation scale next to each day.
2. Ask them to fill it in daily.
3. At the session, review any trends.
4. Discuss ways to address lower-scoring days.

Tips for Debriefing

- Celebrate higher-scoring days or improvements.
- If they forget to log, propose a phone reminder.

Troubleshooting Common Challenges

- If the client sees big swings, explore triggers or supportive actions.
- If they're stuck in low numbers, connect them with resources or reevaluate their approach.

Reflection Questions

- Which day had the biggest slump, and why?
- How might you boost motivation on tough days?

Real life application

Winnie scored her motivation daily, noticing dips on Mondays due to weekend fatigue. She scheduled a short morning walk and uplifting music on Sunday nights, improving her Monday rating.

Worksheet 29: Values and Change Mapping

Title

Values and Change Mapping

The Purpose

You link each stated value (e.g., family, creativity) to the possible benefits of achieving this goal, clarifying alignment between personal ideals and action.

The Rationale

Sheldon and Kasser (1998) emphasise that connecting actions to core values fosters deeper, lasting motivation.

Step-by-Step Instructions

1. Have the client list key values (love, independence, honesty).
2. Next to each, list how the proposed change supports that value.
3. Ask which links feel strongest.
4. Encourage them to recall these connections when temptation to quit arises.

Tips for Debriefing

- Reinforce that seeing a clear link can make daily efforts more meaningful.
- Discuss which value resonates most with them right now.

Troubleshooting Common Challenges

- If no clear link emerges, help them reframe the goal or refine it.
- If multiple values overlap, focus on the top one or two to avoid confusion.

Reflection Questions

- Which value link energises you most?
- How can these connections guide your daily choices?

Real life application
Cal valued honesty and reliability. Realising that controlling his temper let him be more genuine in relationships and keep promises made him more committed to anger management steps.

Worksheet 30: Anticipating Positive Ripple Effects

Title
Anticipating Positive Ripple Effects

The Purpose
You encourage the client to imagine how personal change might benefit friends, family, or colleagues, amplifying their sense of purpose.

The Rationale
Norcross et al. (2011) note that seeing wider impacts can inspire stronger follow-through. Being a force for good can be motivating.

Step-by-Step Instructions

1. List close relationships or areas of life (work, community).
2. For each, ask how success with this goal might help.
3. Encourage them to note intangible gains like increased patience or better mood.
4. Summarise these positive ripples as added incentive.

Tips for Debriefing

- Stress that your client can enrich others by improving themselves.

- Discuss how they might share or celebrate these impacts with loved ones.

Troubleshooting Common Challenges

- If they're self-focused, gently mention how others can be uplifted by their growth.
- If they worry about overshadowing their own needs, reassure them it's a win-win scenario.

Reflection Questions

- Which ripple effect feels most worthwhile?
- How does knowing you'll help others shape your motivation?

Real life application
Sara saw that reducing stress would let her stop snapping at her kids, boosting family harmony. That realisation fueled her to keep using calming techniques daily.

Worksheet 31: Narrative Rewrite

Title
Narrative Rewrite

The Purpose
You invite clients to rewrite a personal story about their struggles, casting themselves as proactive and capable, fostering a more hopeful mindset.

The Rationale
White and Epston (1990) suggest that re-authoring negative scripts can free people from self-defeating labels, promoting fresh perspectives.

Step-by-Step Instructions

1. Pick a past event or pattern they see as a failure.
2. Ask them to rewrite the story focusing on resilience, lessons learned, or small triumphs.

3. Prompt them to read it aloud if comfortable.
4. Reflect how it differs from the old version.

Tips for Debriefing

- Affirm that both versions hold truth but the new angle highlights growth.
- Check if they feel any relief or empowerment.

Troubleshooting Common Challenges

- If they find rewriting awkward, start with bullet points.
- If they revert to blaming themselves, gently remind them of strengths from the story.

Reflection Questions

- Which detail in your new version changes your self-view?
- How can this new perspective guide you moving forward?

Real life application
Adam called himself "a dropout" for leaving college. Reframing, he saw he'd left to support family financially, showing sacrifice and grit. This fresh angle boosted his self-esteem for future studies.

Worksheet 32: Prompting Future Gratitude

Title
Prompting Future Gratitude

The Purpose
You help clients note why their future self might thank them for acting now, reinforcing the notion that today's efforts lead to tomorrow's gratitude.

The Rationale
Emmons and McCullough (2003) show gratitude fosters optimism. Envisioning future thanks can maintain a forward outlook.

Step-by-Step Instructions

1. Ask them to imagine themselves after some months of progress.
2. Write 2–3 reasons their future self says "Thanks for doing that."
3. Reflect on how hearing such appreciation feels.
4. Encourage them to keep these "thank you" notes visible.

Tips for Debriefing

- Normalise any emotional reaction to self-gratitude.
- Link each thank-you reason to a daily habit.

Troubleshooting Common Challenges

- If they're sceptical, treat it as a creative exercise.
- If they have trouble, remind them they'll likely see improvements with consistent effort.

Reflection Questions

- Which reason for future gratitude surprises or touches you most?
- How will you keep these notes in mind day to day?

Real life application
Julia pictured her future self saying, "Thank you for finally getting help for anxiety—I feel calmer, and our relationships are better." Reading this phrase each morning boosted her drive to attend therapy.

Worksheet 33: Fears to Hopes

Title
Fears to Hopes

The Purpose
You ask the client to list worries about change, then actively transform each fear into a hopeful outcome, shifting focus to possibilities.

The Rationale
Lazarus and Folkman (1984) show that reappraising fears as potential wins can lower anxiety and enhance motivation.

Step-by-Step Instructions

1. Write each fear about the upcoming change on one side.
2. Opposite it, create a parallel hope (fear: "I'll fail at this," hope: "I might learn valuable skills").
3. Discuss how reframing might influence mindset.
4. Keep this sheet handy for anxious moments.

Tips for Debriefing

- Validate fears as normal.
- Demonstrate that each fear can hold a positive flip side.

Troubleshooting Common Challenges

- If they can't find a hope for a fear, brainstorm micro-steps or smaller gains.
- If they doubt the reframe, gently ask them to test or imagine it temporarily.

Reflection Questions

- Which fear was hardest to transform into hope?
- How do these new hopes affect your desire to move forward?

Real life application
Josh worried "I'll be miserable without cigarettes." He flipped it to "I might be happier not feeling so dependent." This reframe softened his dread of quitting.

Worksheet 34: Noting Physical Reactions

Title
Noting Physical Reactions

The Purpose
You prompt the client to notice bodily responses (tension, warmth, relief) when discussing change, adding another layer of self-awareness.

The Rationale
Craig (2009) emphasises that physical sensations often accompany emotional shifts. Recognising them can guide better self-regulation.

Step-by-Step Instructions

1. Ask the client to close their eyes or sit quietly.
2. Talk briefly about their desired change, prompting them to observe any bodily sensations.
3. Have them record these feelings (e.g., tight chest, fluttering stomach).
4. Reflect on how these signals might guide or caution them.

Tips for Debriefing

- Remind them it's normal to find both comfort and discomfort.
- Suggest mindful breathing if intense sensations appear.

Troubleshooting Common Challenges

- If they say they feel nothing, gently encourage small details—breath pace, muscle tension.
- If anxiety surfaces, pause for grounding.

Reflection Questions

- What physical signs told you you're excited or nervous?
- How might paying attention to your body help with daily decisions?

Real life application
Celia realised her heart sped up each time she pictured leaving her unfulfilling job. She interpreted that as both fear and excitement, choosing to plan a safer but still intentional career shift.

Worksheet 35: Focused Journaling Exercise

Title
Focused Journaling Exercise

The Purpose
You encourage short, targeted journaling about motivations, mini-wins, or feelings to keep the client connected to their goal.

The Rationale
Pennebaker (1997) suggests that directed writing fosters clarity and self-awareness, aiding steady progress.

Step-by-Step Instructions

1. Assign a simple prompt: "What boosted my motivation today?"
2. Ask them to jot down a few sentences each evening.
3. Review entries at sessions to note patterns or surprises.
4. Adjust the prompt as needed for variety.

Tips for Debriefing

- Praise consistency if they stick with daily writing.
- If they skip days, reassure them it's okay; pick up whenever possible.

Troubleshooting Common Challenges

- If they don't like writing, consider voice memos or quick bullet points.
- If journaling evokes strong emotions, offer gentle support and boundaries.

Reflection Questions

- Which recurring theme do you see in your entries?
- How does noting daily motivations affect your drive?

Real life application
Arun recorded small triumphs each night ("Managed to avoid negative self-talk at

work"). After a week, he felt encouraged by the daily logs, seeing progress building slowly.

Worksheet 36: Prompting Specific Steps

Title
Prompting Specific Steps

The Purpose
You transform vague intentions into clear, measurable actions, helping your client see exactly what to do next.

The Rationale
Doran (1981) introduced SMART principles. Being specific fosters better follow-through and less procrastination.

Step-by-Step Instructions

1. Listen for a client's general statement like "I want to eat healthier."
2. Ask, "How exactly can you do that?"
3. Brainstorm an actionable task: "Buy vegetables every Sunday and cook them twice a week."
4. Encourage them to confirm they feel ready to attempt it.

Tips for Debriefing

- Keep goals small at first.
- Link the action step to their main motivation.

Troubleshooting Common Challenges

- If they resist narrowing it down, highlight the benefits of tangible steps.
- If it's still too broad, help them set times, places, or amounts.

Reflection Questions

- Which specific action do you feel confident about?
- How soon will you start?

Real life application
Dean's "I should exercise more" became "I'll take a 15-minute walk after lunch on weekdays." That clarity made him stick to the plan more effectively.

Worksheet 37: Discussing Role Models

Title
Discussing Role Models

The Purpose
You return to the idea of individuals who overcame a similar issue, gleaning practical or moral support from their journey.

The Rationale
Lockwood et al. (2005) indicate that looking to successful peers or public figures can reaffirm that change is possible.

Step-by-Step Instructions

1. Invite them to revisit or find a new role model.
2. Write down qualities, steps, or attitudes that led to success.
3. Reflect on how each can be adapted.
4. Note which part of the role model's approach they find most doable.

Tips for Debriefing

- Remind them they can combine different role models' strengths.
- Encourage curiosity rather than direct copying.

Troubleshooting Common Challenges

- If a client idolises someone unrealistic, guide them to see the human side of that model.

- If they feel envy, discuss how that can be turned into inspiration.

Reflection Questions

- What new lesson did you discover from this role model?
- How might you apply that lesson this week?

Real life application
Kim admired a friend who overcame social shyness by volunteering at a local shelter, building confidence through service. Kim decided to join a nearby charity group to expand her social comfort zone.

Worksheet 38: Comparing Outcomes

Title
Comparing Outcomes

The Purpose
You place immediate gains versus future rewards side by side, emphasising how today's efforts can yield greater benefits later on.

The Rationale
Ariely and Wertenbroch (2002) illustrate that acknowledging future payoffs can make short-term sacrifices more palatable.

Step-by-Step Instructions

1. Create two columns: "Immediate Gains" vs. "Future Gains."
2. Ask them to fill each with potential positives of making this change, focusing on time horizons.
3. Discuss if the long-term gains overshadow any short-lived struggles.
4. Let them reflect on which column sparks more commitment.

Tips for Debriefing

- Highlight how short-term sacrifices can be stepping stones.

- Validate that immediate comforts can be hard to give up.

Troubleshooting Common Challenges

- If they're fixated on instant gratification, remind them of the reasons that matter more over time.
- If future rewards feel too distant, propose short "wins" along the journey.

Reflection Questions

- Which long-term benefit feels most motivating?
- How do these columns influence your priorities?

Real life application
Casey placed "extra free time" under Immediate Gains for skipping study. Under Future Gains, she listed "passing exams, career growth." Realising the future gains were key, she trimmed her leisure hours slightly to study more.

Worksheet 39: Public Commitment

Title
Public Commitment

The Purpose
You invite clients comfortable with going public to declare their goal to friends, family, or a group, reinforcing accountability.

The Rationale
Cialdini and Goldstein (2004) show that public promises often bolster consistency, as people wish to follow through on stated aims.

Step-by-Step Instructions

1. Ask who they trust enough to share their aim.
2. Discuss the preferred method: a social media post, an email, or telling close friends.

3. Encourage them to set a timeline for that announcement.
4. Explore how support or occasional check-ins might help.

Tips for Debriefing

- Stress picking an encouraging audience.
- If they prefer privacy, remind them that minimal sharing can still be powerful.

Troubleshooting Common Challenges

- If they fear judgement, reassure them that supportive feedback is key.
- If they have no supportive network, consider a small online forum or buddy system.

Reflection Questions

- How do you feel about making your goal public?
- What kind of response would help most?

Real life application
Brenda posted online that she was committing to a month of alcohol-free living. The supportive comments and occasional queries about her progress kept her on track, even when cravings hit.

Worksheet 40: Reflection Celebration

Title
Reflection Celebration

The Purpose
You wrap up by recounting your client's strongest change statements or successes, honouring their resolve and setting the stage for next steps.

The Rationale
Miller and Rollnick (2013) highlight that concluding on a note of positivity and clarity cements motivation and fosters continuity.

Step-by-Step Instructions

1. Near session's end, recall any powerful statements the client made about changing.
2. Reflect them back with emphasis on their words.
3. Invite the client to comment on how it feels hearing them again.
4. Affirm progress, and encourage them to use these phrases until the next meeting.

Tips for Debriefing

- Applaud even minor signs of progress.
- Suggest they jot down these strong statements for daily reference.

Troubleshooting Common Challenges

- If the client dismisses praise, reinforce the sincerity of your reflections.
- If they ended the session on a low note, try to highlight even a small positive statement.

Reflection Questions

- Which statement or success do you feel proudest of?
- How can you keep this momentum going after today?

Real life application

At the close, Pam heard her words repeated: "I've decided my health can't wait." She felt inspired listening to her own conviction and left more confident in her plan to exercise thrice weekly.

Reflective Listening and Communication

Worksheets here refine your ability to paraphrase and reflect the client's statements, capturing both facts and emotions. This deeper level of listening strengthens understanding and encourages clients to elaborate. It also fosters a calmer atmosphere for insightful, empathic discussions.

Worksheet 1: Four Levels of Reflection

Title
Four Levels of Reflection

The Purpose
You develop skills to move from repeating a client's words to offering reflections about deeper emotions and meaning. This approach enriches conversations and allows the client to feel understood.

The Rationale
Rogers (1957) indicates that reflective listening in layers—starting with repetition and moving toward deeper interpretations—helps clients explore hidden feelings. By showing empathy at each level, you strengthen rapport and encourage more open sharing.

Step-by-Step Instructions

1. Prepare four categories: Simple Repetition, Paraphrase, Reflection of Feeling, Reflection of Meaning.
2. Listen to a client statement. Write it down or mentally note it.
3. Try reflecting at each level, from simply echoing their words to capturing the unspoken significance.
4. Notice which level resonates or elicits further detail from the client.

Tips for Debriefing

- Ask the client which reflection style felt most accurate.
- Emphasise that deeper levels need care and should be offered gently.

Troubleshooting Common Challenges

- If deeper reflections feel uncomfortable, practise with shorter statements first.
- If the client corrects you, let them shape the reflection until it feels right.

Reflection Questions

- Which level brought the most insight?

- How can you become more comfortable offering deeper reflections?

Real life application
A counsellor first repeated a client's phrase word for word. Then they paraphrased it, acknowledged the emotion, and finally saw a deeper belief about the client's fear of rejection. This four-step process revealed valuable insight.

Worksheet 2: Matching Emotional Tone

Title
Matching Emotional Tone

The Purpose
You learn to notice and reflect the client's emotional intensity, ensuring your response aligns with their feelings instead of overlooking them.

The Rationale
Hill (2010) points out that mirroring the client's emotional level fosters safety. If you underreact or overreact, they may feel misunderstood or overwhelmed.

Step-by-Step Instructions

1. Observe the client's voice, speed, and body language.
2. Reflect back their words using a similar level of energy or calmness.
3. Check the client's reaction to see if you matched them well.
4. Adjust if you sense discomfort or if they correct your interpretation.

Tips for Debriefing

- If they're low energy, respond softly; if they're excited, show corresponding enthusiasm.
- Subtle shifts in your tone can make them feel heard.

Troubleshooting Common Challenges

- If you mimic them too strongly, they might feel parodied. Keep it gentle.

- If you sense a mismatch, simply apologise and adapt your approach.

Reflection Questions

- How did matching their tone affect trust or openness?
- Did you notice any difference in the depth of their sharing?

Real life application
A therapist realised her client spoke in a hushed voice, revealing sadness. By lowering her own voice and reflecting the sadness, the therapist saw the client open up further, feeling validated.

Worksheet 3: Reframing Statement

Title
Reframing Statement

The Purpose
You learn to take a client's negative or harsh self-talk and reflect it with a focus on strengths or a more balanced viewpoint, reducing self-blame.

The Rationale
Beck (2011) shows that reframing negative beliefs boosts hope. Guiding clients to see possibilities instead of failures can encourage them to keep going.

Step-by-Step Instructions

1. Listen for a self-critical remark (e.g., "I'm useless at everything").
2. Reflect it back, but shift the lens: "You might feel defeated now, yet you managed to reach out for help."
3. Check if this kinder perspective resonates.
4. Encourage the client to adopt a balanced view of their challenges.

Tips for Debriefing

- Highlight real examples of the client's effort or good qualities.

- Avoid denying their feelings; gently offer a fresh angle.

Troubleshooting Common Challenges

- If they resist the reframe, ask about a smaller success they might accept.
- Ensure you're sincere, not just cheering them up blindly.

Reflection Questions

- Which part of the reframed statement feels true?
- How could you reframe your thoughts in daily life?

Real life application

Leslie said, "I always mess up." The therapist reframed, pointing out past times Leslie solved problems effectively. Leslie felt relief, seeing she wasn't a total failure.

Worksheet 4: Reflecting Content vs. Emotion

Title

Reflecting Content vs. Emotion

The Purpose

You practise deciding when to emphasise the client's factual details and when to highlight their feelings. Balancing both can deepen mutual understanding.

The Rationale

Rogers (1957) found that tuning in to both facts and emotions creates a more complete reflection. Sometimes a client needs clarity on events; other times they need validation of how they feel.

Step-by-Step Instructions

1. Ask the client to describe a recent event.
2. First, reflect the event's content (who, what, when).
3. Then reflect any implied emotions (anger, sadness, excitement).
4. Discuss which style helps them feel most understood.

Tips for Debriefing

- Ask for feedback on whether they prefer more factual or emotional reflections at different moments.
- Consider the client's emotional state; reflecting feelings can be powerful but also delicate.

Troubleshooting Common Challenges

- If they want practical solutions, focusing too long on feelings may frustrate them.
- If they need to vent emotions, repeating just details might feel cold.

Reflection Questions

- Which reflection (content or emotion) resonated more with you?
- How does blending both approaches help you process the situation?

Real life application
Matthew described a fight at home. The therapist first repeated the sequence of events. Then they acknowledged Matthew's sense of betrayal and pain. He appreciated hearing both sides recognised.

Worksheet 5: Behind the Words

Title
Behind the Words

The Purpose
You sharpen your ability to pick up on clues that point to deeper concerns. This helps you reflect unspoken feelings, inviting the client to share more fully.

The Rationale
Egan (2013) notes that clients often give subtle hints about deeper issues. Naming these clues in a reflection can unlock more honest discussion.

Step-by-Step Instructions

1. During conversation, listen for tone shifts, body language, or repeated phrases.
2. Reflect possible underlying emotions: "I sense you might be frustrated, not just annoyed?"
3. Wait to see if they correct or confirm you.
4. Explore that deeper layer if they agree.

Tips for Debriefing

- Approach with curiosity rather than certainty.
- Encourage the client to clarify if your reflection doesn't feel right.

Troubleshooting Common Challenges

- If they dismiss your guess, simply thank them for clarifying.
- If they show distress, ensure they feel safe stepping back or changing topics.

Reflection Questions

- Did noticing subtle hints reveal any new perspective?
- How can you become more attentive to nonverbal signals?

Real life application

Connie often used sarcasm about her workload. The therapist gently reflected, "It sounds like there's stress behind that humour." Connie admitted she felt unappreciated, leading to deeper exploration.

Worksheet 6: Pitfalls in Reflective Listening

Title

Pitfalls in Reflective Listening

The Purpose

You identify and address common mistakes—like sounding fake or overusing certain phrases—that hinder effective listening.

The Rationale

Swift et al. (2017) mention that awareness of errors like parroting or minimising helps you avoid them. Correcting these habits can strengthen trust.

Step-by-Step Instructions

1. List potential pitfalls: repeating words robotically, interrupting, offering solutions too soon, oversimplifying feelings.
2. Check which you might fall into.
3. Brainstorm ways to avoid each pitfall (e.g., limit how often you say "It sounds like…").
4. Practise mindful listening, watching for slip-ups.

Tips for Debriefing

- Remind yourself that improvement is a gradual process.
- If you notice a pitfall mid-session, it's fine to course-correct immediately.

Troubleshooting Common Challenges

- If you catch yourself using filler phrases repeatedly, try pausing before speaking.
- If you interrupt, practise waiting a breath or two after the client finishes talking.

Reflection Questions

- Which pitfall do you most often slip into?
- How might changing that habit enhance client comfort?

Real life application

Marina, a new therapist, realised she repeatedly said, "So you feel…" in a monotone way. She began varying her language and tone, and clients responded more warmly.

Worksheet 7: Listening to Empower

Title
Listening to Empower

The Purpose
You fine-tune reflections that underscore a client's strengths or capabilities, helping them view themselves as resourceful and resilient.

The Rationale
Seligman (2011) shows that highlighting assets encourages a positive outlook. Clients who feel competent tend to make braver decisions.

Step-by-Step Instructions

1. Listen for any success, big or small, in their story.
2. Reflect it back: "That shows real dedication," or "You handled a tricky situation calmly."
3. Check how they respond. Ask how they might use this strength elsewhere.
4. Build a list of qualities they recognise in themselves.

Tips for Debriefing

- Keep your tone genuine, avoiding forced compliments.
- Link the strength to their current goal, e.g., "Your patience might help you cope with stress."

Troubleshooting Common Challenges

- If they dismiss praise, offer specific evidence ("You worked late to finish the project").
- If no obvious strengths appear, look for small steps or attempts they made.

Reflection Questions

- Which strengths do you feel proud of now?
- How can these strengths support future challenges?

Real life application
Kevin often belittled himself at work. The therapist reflected, "Staying late to solve that error shows persistence." Kevin realised he wasn't lazy but consistently tried hard.

Worksheet 8: Double-Check Reflections

Title
Double-Check Reflections

The Purpose
You confirm accuracy by inviting the client to modify or expand on your reflection, preventing misunderstandings and refining empathy.

The Rationale
Hill (2010) suggests that checking in after a reflection ensures the client feels heard correctly, building trust in the conversation.

Step-by-Step Instructions

1. Reflect a client's statement: "You're worried about letting your team down."
2. Ask, "Does that ring true, or is there more to it?"
3. Listen as they confirm or adjust your words.
4. Integrate their clarification to refine your reflection.

Tips for Debriefing

- Show appreciation for any correction, viewing it as teamwork.
- Use short questions like, "Did I get that right?" to keep the flow.

Troubleshooting Common Challenges

- If they simply say "Yes," gently prompt them to elaborate.
- If they disagree, thank them and reflect their new statement.

Reflection Questions

- How does checking in help you avoid assumptions?
- Did you notice a difference in how they opened up after confirming?

Real life application
Marissa reflected, "It seems like you're frustrated with your boss," then asked for accuracy. Her client said it was more disappointment than anger, revealing a new emotion that guided deeper conversation.

Worksheet 9: Complex Reflection Practice

Title
Complex Reflection Practice

The Purpose
You merge factual and emotional layers in the same reflection, aiming for a richer response that captures multiple dimensions of the client's experience.

The Rationale
Miller and Rollnick (2013) highlight that deeper reflections—combining content and feelings—can lead to significant insights.

Step-by-Step Instructions

1. Pick a brief client statement describing an event ("I argued with my sister all night.").
2. Reflect both what happened and how they felt: "You argued with her for hours, and it left you feeling annoyed and let down."
3. Observe their reaction or elaboration.
4. Fine-tune your reflection if they add more context.

Tips for Debriefing

- Keep the statement concise yet comprehensive.
- Ensure you balance factual detail with the emotional undertone.

Troubleshooting Common Challenges

- If the client says you missed a key detail, revise your reflection.

- If they only confirm factual points, gently probe for how it impacted them emotionally.

Reflection Questions

- How did this fuller reflection change the discussion?
- Did you learn anything new about the client's viewpoint?

Real life application

Sarah mentioned a tense evening with her daughter. The therapist acknowledged both the repeated disagreements and Sarah's sense of sadness, prompting Sarah to discuss underlying worries about losing closeness.

Worksheet 10: Using Silence to Reflect

Title
Using Silence to Reflect

The Purpose
You practise offering a reflection, then pausing briefly to let the client absorb it, revealing deeper layers of their thoughts.

The Rationale
Hill (2010) observes that thoughtful silence encourages clients to reflect further. A slight pause often prompts them to share more insight.

Step-by-Step Instructions

1. Reflect a client statement succinctly: "You're feeling uncertain about your next step."
2. Stop talking for a few seconds.
3. Notice if they continue or process your words.
4. If they remain silent, gently ask, "Is there anything more on your mind?"

Tips for Debriefing

- Resist filling the pause too quickly.
- Show supportive nonverbal cues (soft eye contact, nod).

Troubleshooting Common Challenges

- If they get uncomfortable, explain that silence is a chance to reflect, not a sign of disapproval.
- If they never resume speaking, ask a brief follow-up question.

Reflection Questions

- How did silence affect the depth of the conversation?
- Did they reveal anything extra during that quiet moment?

Real life application
Tom gave a short answer about feeling "off." The therapist reflected that comment and went quiet. Tom soon elaborated on deeper insecurities he'd never mentioned before.

Worksheet 11: Transitional Reflections

Title
Transitional Reflections

The Purpose
You help the conversation flow smoothly when shifting from one topic to another, using statements that link ideas without abrupt changes.

The Rationale
Miller and Rollnick (2013) mention that bridging reflections keep the client feeling heard. They also maintain momentum if multiple concerns arise.

Step-by-Step Instructions

1. Summarise the current topic: "We've explored your work stress."
2. Gently introduce the next theme: "It also sounds like that stress influences your sleep."

3. Invite the client to confirm or correct the link.
4. Transition at their pace, allowing them to linger if needed.

Tips for Debriefing

- If they want to stay on the old topic longer, respect that.
- Use transitional phrases sparingly, ensuring each shift feels natural.

Troubleshooting Common Challenges

- If they resist shifting, reflect that reluctance: "You're not ready to move on yet."
- If the new topic is sensitive, proceed with caution and empathy.

Reflection Questions

- Did linking the two topics help you see a bigger picture?
- Which transitions felt seamless?

Real life application
Carla discussed her insomnia and her anxiety. The therapist used a transitional reflection: "So we've covered your anxiety at work, and it's affecting your sleep. Shall we explore your bedtime routine next?" Carla found it a logical step.

Worksheet 12: Mirroring Body Language

Title
Mirroring Body Language

The Purpose
You subtly mirror a client's posture or movements, fostering rapport and showing that you're in tune with them.

The Rationale
Koole and Tschacher (2016) note that gentle mimicry can enhance empathy and trust, though it should never be forced.

Step-by-Step Instructions

1. Observe the client's posture—are they leaning forward, sitting back, hands clasped?
2. Gently adopt a similar stance or position.
3. If they shift, you might shift after a short pause.
4. See if they relax or open up as a result.

Tips for Debriefing

- Keep your mirroring subtle; don't copy every gesture.
- If they seem self-conscious, ease off and stick to reflective listening verbally.

Troubleshooting Common Challenges

- If they notice and joke about it, calmly mention you're aiming for comfort.
- If it feels unnatural, don't push it—some clients prefer just verbal empathy.

Reflection Questions

- How did matching their posture affect the energy in the room?
- Did they speak more freely as a result?

Real life application
John sat slightly forward with folded arms. The therapist matched that stance lightly. Over time, John unfolded his arms and seemed calmer, prompting deeper sharing.

Worksheet 13: Balancing Affirmation and Reflection

Title
Balancing Affirmation and Reflection

The Purpose
You practise weaving together compliments about the client's strengths with reflective statements, validating both their abilities and emotions.

The Rationale

Miller and Rollnick (2013) state that affirmations boost self-esteem, while reflections ensure clients feel understood. Together, they can bolster hope and openness.

Step-by-Step Instructions

1. Listen for any positive aspect—a client's perseverance, creativity, or courage.
2. Affirm it: "That shows determination."
3. Follow with a reflective statement of their feelings or perspective.
4. Note how this combination influences their emotional state.

Tips for Debriefing

- Aim for specificity: "You overcame that big hurdle," not just "Great job."
- Ensure the reflection addresses emotional or factual details.

Troubleshooting Common Challenges

- Overemphasising compliments could seem insincere if there's no reflection.
- If they reject praise, remind them why you see their efforts as noteworthy.

Reflection Questions

- Did affirmation plus reflection feel balanced to you?
- How might this blend encourage more discussion?

Real life application

Diana shared her daily walk goal. The therapist affirmed her commitment, then reflected her slight worry about time constraints. This mix made Diana feel both seen and encouraged.

Worksheet 14: Short vs. Extended Reflections

Title

Short vs. Extended Reflections

The Purpose
You decide when a concise reflection is enough and when a more thorough reflection is helpful, adapting your approach to each moment.

The Rationale
Hill (2010) mentions that brief reflections often clarify small points, while extended ones uncover deeper layers.

Step-by-Step Instructions

1. Practise responding to simple statements with a short reflection: "You felt disappointed."
2. For more charged or multifaceted statements, offer an extended version: "You tried your best and still felt let down, which is really upsetting."
3. Ask which style resonates better with the client in that situation.

Tips for Debriefing

- Observe the client's reaction. If a short reflection leaves them hanging, try a more expansive one.
- If time is limited, keep it concise.

Troubleshooting Common Challenges

- If you always offer long reflections, the client may get overwhelmed.
- If you remain too brief, they might sense you're not fully engaged.

Reflection Questions

- When does a short response suffice?
- What clues suggest you need a deeper reflection?

Real life application
Allison was venting about her partner's neglect. A short reflection "You feel ignored" wasn't enough. The therapist added, "You put in effort yet feel your partner isn't reciprocating, leaving you hurt," which prompted Allison to open up further.

Worksheet 15: Responding to Resistant Statements

Title
Responding to Resistant Statements

The Purpose
You soften pushback by reflecting the client's reluctance without arguing, helping them feel heard while opening room for change.

The Rationale
Miller and Rollnick (2013) explain that acknowledging resistance calmly defuses defensiveness and invites conversation rather than conflict.

Step-by-Step Instructions

1. Listen for signs of resistance: "I don't see why I should do this."
2. Reflect back: "You're doubtful about the benefit here."
3. Wait to see if they explain further or modify their stance.
4. Maintain empathy without insisting they must change.

Tips for Debriefing

- Keep your voice calm and respectful.
- Recognise the client's autonomy to accept or reject advice.

Troubleshooting Common Challenges

- If they grow more resistant, reflect their frustration: "You feel forced into this."
- If they demand immediate solutions, gently keep exploring their perspective first.

Reflection Questions

- How did reflecting their resistance shift the tension?
- Did they share more once you accepted their doubts?

Real life application
Grace insisted therapy was pointless. The therapist replied, "You're not convinced this

226

can help." Grace softened, elaborating that she'd tried similar help before with no results, opening a path to discuss fresh approaches.

Worksheet 16: Experimenting with Emphasis

Title
Experimenting with Emphasis

The Purpose
You reflect back a client's words but shift which word or phrase you stress, seeing if it draws out deeper meanings or corrections.

The Rationale
Discourse analysis (Gee, 2014) shows that altering emphasis can highlight hidden layers. Clients often clarify or realise nuances they hadn't shared openly.

Step-by-Step Instructions

1. Pick a short client statement: "I just can't stand my job."
2. Reflect it, each time stressing a different word: "You CAN'T stand your job?" / "You can't STAND your job?"
3. Note the client's response, whether they correct or expand.
4. Ask them to confirm which emphasis feels most accurate.

Tips for Debriefing

- Use this skill sparingly so it doesn't seem forced.
- Watch body language to gauge if it reveals new insights.

Troubleshooting Common Challenges

- If they become annoyed, explain you're clarifying meaning.
- If it yields nothing, switch to a different listening technique.

Reflection Questions

- Which emphasis did you find gave new insight?
- How did focusing on different words change your understanding?

Real life application
Finn said, "I'm so tired of this routine." The therapist echoed, "You're SO tired?" prompting Finn to realise it wasn't just a minor bother—he felt truly drained daily.

Worksheet 17: Summarizing Big Themes

Title
Summarizing Big Themes

The Purpose
You periodically gather the key ideas or emotions discussed, ensuring coherence and helping the client see patterns in their story.

The Rationale
Miller and Rollnick (2013) suggest summarising main points confirms understanding and can reveal insights about repeated struggles or hopes.

Step-by-Step Instructions

1. After a section of discussion, pause to recap: "You're worried about finances, and it's causing tension at home."
2. Include the feelings you heard: "That tension makes you feel anxious and drained."
3. Check if the client wants to add or clarify.
4. Use the summary to shift toward problem-solving or next steps.

Tips for Debriefing

- Keep your summary brief but thorough.
- Notice if summarising triggers a new realisation for the client.

Troubleshooting Common Challenges

- If they say you missed something, incorporate it at once.
- If they're bored by summaries, keep them concise or less frequent.

Reflection Questions

- Did hearing the main points help you see an overall pattern?
- Which theme resonates most strongly?

Real life application
Paula discussed financial strain, relationship stress, and guilt about not supporting her parents. The therapist summarised these themes, prompting Paula to link everything to her fear of letting people down.

Worksheet 18: Reflective Listening Drills

Title
Reflective Listening Drills

The Purpose
You enhance your listening by practising reflection with short mock scenarios or real client statements, receiving feedback to refine your approach.

The Rationale
Hill (2010) states that repetition in low-pressure drills cements reflective habits, making them more natural in actual sessions.

Step-by-Step Instructions

1. Gather sample client statements ("I hate my job," "I feel alone").
2. Respond with a reflection, focusing on emotion or meaning.
3. If practising with a colleague, let them critique clarity and empathy.
4. Adjust phrasing, tone, or content until it feels genuine.

Tips for Debriefing

- Keep the setting supportive.

- Record attempts (audio or notes) to track improvements.

Troubleshooting Common Challenges

- If you feel awkward, start with simpler statements.
- If feedback stings, remember it's part of growing your skills.

Reflection Questions

- Which statements did you find toughest to reflect?
- How can you bring more warmth or accuracy next time?

Real life application
Juan tested reflective responses on statements like "I'm so stressed." Over a few drills, he learned to better capture both the frustration and underlying fear, resulting in more heartfelt reflections.

Worksheet 19: Capturing Client Language

Title
Capturing Client Language

The Purpose
You practise echoing a client's key words or phrases exactly, honouring their unique expression and helping them feel genuinely heard.

The Rationale
Elliott et al. (2011) note that using a client's own phrasing can deepen trust. Hearing familiar words back signals you truly listen.

Step-by-Step Instructions

1. Listen for distinctive words the client uses.
2. Reflect them verbatim: "So you felt 'drained and stuck' after that meeting."
3. Avoid altering their wording too much.
4. Observe whether it resonates or leads to clarifications.

Tips for Debriefing

- If their words are harsh or explicit, still echo them gently unless it disrupts safety.
- Acknowledge any cultural or personal significance in certain phrases.

Troubleshooting Common Challenges

- If you feel uneasy repeating strong language, maintain sincerity while respecting your own comfort.
- If they use a term you don't understand, ask for meaning or context.

Reflection Questions

- Did reflecting their exact words prompt more openness?
- Which phrases were most revealing?

Real life application

Chris repeatedly used "I'm stuck in a dead-end." The therapist said, "You keep calling it a 'dead-end'—that must feel hopeless." Chris then explained exactly why he felt no escape, guiding a more focused discussion.

Worksheet 20: Encouraging Deeper Elaboration

Title
Encouraging Deeper Elaboration

The Purpose
You add an open-ended follow-up after a reflection, giving clients an opportunity to expand and access greater insight.

The Rationale
Hill (2010) reports that pairing reflection with a gentle invitation to say more often uncovers underlying details.

Step-by-Step Instructions

1. Reflect the client's words.
2. Immediately follow up with, "Could you tell me more about that?" or "What else was going on?"
3. Wait while they think, maintaining interest.
4. Reflect again if new content emerges.

Tips for Debriefing

- Avoid peppering them with too many questions at once.
- Show you're genuinely curious, not interrogating.

Troubleshooting Common Challenges

- If they say "That's all," respect their boundary.
- If they feel rushed, slow your pace or give them a moment of quiet.

Reflection Questions

- Which elaboration revealed something unexpected?
- How did it feel to invite more detail?

Real life application
Nate said he felt anxious about an upcoming exam. The therapist replied, "You sound worried and pressured—could you say more about what makes it feel so intense?" Nate then admitted he feared letting his parents down, a core issue.

Worksheet 21: Reflective Listening Journal

Title
Reflective Listening Journal

The Purpose
You record and review your reflective attempts after each session, reinforcing strong points and noticing areas to enhance.

The Rationale

Schön (1983) suggests that systematic reflection on one's practice fosters continuous improvement. Tracking your reflections sharpens your listening skills over time.

Step-by-Step Instructions

1. After each session, jot down 1–2 reflections you offered.
2. Note what worked well and any challenging moments.
3. Plan one small adjustment or goal for the next session.
4. Revisit these journal entries to watch your growth.

Tips for Debriefing

- Keep it brief so it remains a habit.
- Periodically share insights with a supervisor or peer for added input.

Troubleshooting Common Challenges

- If you forget, set a reminder immediately after sessions.
- If you overanalyse, limit each entry to key highlights.

Reflection Questions

- How did reviewing your reflections guide your next approach?
- Which repeating pattern did you spot?

Real life application

Serena logged reflections daily. She noticed she often used a bright tone even when clients were sad. Realising this mismatch, she learned to lower her tone when reflecting sadness, making clients feel more seen.

Worksheet 22: Acknowledge Contradictions

Title

Acknowledge Contradictions

The Purpose
You highlight inconsistencies when a client's statements conflict, reflecting both sides gently without shaming them.

The Rationale
Linehan (1993) shows that spotting contradictions helps clients confront ambivalence. Pointing this out kindly can spark clarity or resolution.

Step-by-Step Instructions

1. Pick up on two conflicting remarks (e.g., "I want more independence" and "I wish someone would just fix it for me.").
2. Reflect both: "You want to stand on your own, yet a part of you craves direct help."
3. Ask them how it feels to hold both views.
4. Invite exploration of any next steps or solutions.

Tips for Debriefing

- Normalise having mixed feelings.
- Maintain a calm tone to prevent defensiveness.

Troubleshooting Common Challenges

- If they resent your observation, clarify you understand confusion is natural.
- If contradictions remain unresolved, let them stay for now if the client needs more time.

Reflection Questions

- How does seeing both sides laid out affect your perspective?
- What might reconcile these opposing feelings?

Real life application
Marco said he liked solitude yet also felt lonely. The therapist reflected this contradiction. Marco then admitted fear of rejection plus a need for closeness, opening a path to discuss balanced social contact.

Worksheet 23: Reflecting Change Talk

Title
Reflecting Change Talk

The Purpose
You respond promptly to any sign of willingness or desire to change, underscoring its importance and nurturing the client's motivation.

The Rationale
Miller and Rollnick (2013) observe that reinforcing even small statements about wanting change helps clients move from thinking to doing.

Step-by-Step Instructions

1. Listen for key words: "I should," "I want," "I might."
2. Reflect it: "It sounds like you're ready to try something new."
3. Encourage them to build on that idea: "What would be your first step?"
4. Notice if more detailed plans emerge.

Tips for Debriefing

- Celebrate any sign of positivity or intent.
- Keep momentum by asking about specifics once they confirm readiness.

Troubleshooting Common Challenges

- If they backpedal, gently reflect the new hesitation.
- If they say it casually, emphasise its significance to them.

Reflection Questions

- Which change talk statement felt strongest?
- How did reflecting it influence their motivation?

Real life application
Angela said, "I might cut down on sugar." The therapist replied, "You're thinking it's time to make that shift," nudging Angela to plan how to reduce sweets.

Worksheet 24: Focusing on Positive Emotions

Title
Focusing on Positive Emotions

The Purpose
You reflect bright feelings like hope or excitement that a client expresses, reinforcing them so the client recognises and values these emotions.

The Rationale
Fredrickson (2001) highlights that emphasising positive states expands a sense of possibility, helping clients see change as achievable.

Step-by-Step Instructions

1. Tune in when they mention relief, excitement, pride, or joy.
2. Reflect it clearly: "You sound genuinely proud of yourself."
3. Ask them to elaborate on what that pride means.
4. Link the positive emotion to their efforts or strengths.

Tips for Debriefing

- Validate that positive feelings deserve as much attention as negative ones.
- Encourage them to use these moments as motivation anchors.

Troubleshooting Common Challenges

- If they downplay their joy, gently remind them why it's worth celebrating.
- If they rarely show positive emotions, highlight even small glimpses of hope.

Reflection Questions

- How did naming your positive emotion help you appreciate it more?
- Can these good feelings fuel your next steps?

Real life application
Devon beamed when talking about his daily painting routine. The therapist mirrored that excitement and asked, "What does feeling so happy tell you about painting's impact on your life?" This spurred Devon to commit to painting more often.

Worksheet 25: Depth of Empathy

Title
Depth of Empathy

The Purpose
You deepen your reflections by considering the client's worldview—past experiences, culture, beliefs—and empathising beyond surface statements.

The Rationale
Rogers (1957) clarifies that deeper empathy involves stepping into the client's perspective, fostering trust and genuine understanding.

Step-by-Step Instructions

1. Listen not only to words but to context—how might family background or past trauma shape this story?
2. Reflect with references to these contexts: "It makes sense you'd feel anxious, given how your family handled conflict."
3. Notice if they feel recognised or correct your assumptions.
4. Adjust your reflections as they provide more details.

Tips for Debriefing

- Remain humble; you're learning their perspective, not claiming to know it perfectly.
- If uncertain, ask permission to mention cultural or personal factors.

Troubleshooting Common Challenges

- If they bristle at referencing background, simply apologise and let them guide.

- If they appreciate it, keep weaving in relevant contexts.

Reflection Questions

- Did referencing deeper factors resonate or help you feel heard?
- How can you ensure you stay respectful of their personal history?

Real life application

A client felt shame about showing emotions, partly due to a strict upbringing. The therapist reflected, "No wonder you hide your feelings—your background taught you to be stoic," prompting the client to talk about wanting to unlearn that constraint.

Worksheet 26: Reflecting Fear and Doubt

Title

Reflecting Fear and Doubt

The Purpose

You acknowledge a client's hesitations or anxieties without trying to fix them immediately, allowing those feelings to surface safely.

The Rationale

Miller and Rollnick (2013) note that validating worry fosters acceptance. Clients often relax and explore solutions after feeling heard.

Step-by-Step Instructions

1. Hear their concern: "I'm scared I won't succeed."
2. Reflect it plainly: "That fear is heavy for you, especially around success."
3. Ask if there's more to that fear.
4. Let them clarify or deepen the explanation.

Tips for Debriefing

- Show empathy without rushing to solve it.
- Affirm it's natural to have doubts during change.

Troubleshooting Common Challenges

- If fear intensifies, ensure they have coping strategies to calm anxiety.
- If they deny the fear, gently check if they sense any worry in smaller ways.

Reflection Questions

- How does naming your fear help you handle it?
- What step feels safe enough to take despite the doubt?

Real life application

Rita confessed, "I'm scared of failing again." The therapist said, "That fear feels big, especially since you've tried before and got disappointed." Rita sighed, relieved someone understood her anxiety, and then talked about supportive measures to reduce that fear.

Worksheet 27: Breaking Down Defensive Walls

Title
Breaking Down Defensive Walls

The Purpose
You respond to defensiveness by reflecting its root, preventing arguments and fostering curiosity. This can open dialogue about deeper issues.

The Rationale
Rogers (1957) shows that empathic acceptance lowers defensive responses. When clients feel you understand their stance, they become less guarded.

Step-by-Step Instructions

1. When the client seems defensive, reflect, "It sounds like you really want to protect yourself right now."
2. Pause, waiting to see if they drop the defensive tone.
3. Offer reassurance that you respect their perspective.
4. Explore underlying worries or fears once they relax.

Tips for Debriefing

- Maintain calm eye contact if culturally appropriate.
- Affirm you hear their frustration or suspicion.

Troubleshooting Common Challenges

- If they escalate, slow down and affirm their feelings again.
- If you sense hostility, consider small breaks or grounding techniques.

Reflection Questions

- How did reflecting the root of defensiveness help you feel safer?
- Which deeper issue showed up after the initial wall softened?

Real life application
Ben snapped, "You can't understand my situation." The therapist reflected, "You feel misunderstood and don't trust easily." Acknowledging his mistrust allowed him to elaborate on past betrayals, shifting from anger to explanation.

Worksheet 28: Addressing the Unspoken

Title
Addressing the Unspoken

The Purpose
You notice unspoken cues—silence, body language, subtle expressions—and reflect them tentatively. This invites the client to reveal deeper truths they haven't verbalised.

The Rationale
Mehrabian (1972) highlights that much communication is nonverbal. Identifying unspoken tension or emotion encourages clients to share underlying issues.

Step-by-Step Instructions

1. Observe if the client hesitates, avoids eye contact, or sighs.

2. Offer a gentle reflection: "You paused; maybe there's something difficult to express?"
3. Wait for a response, letting them fill in details if they choose.
4. Reassure them it's safe to speak openly or correct your impression.

Tips for Debriefing

- Keep your voice soft, ensuring they feel no pressure.
- If they deny anything, let it go politely.

Troubleshooting Common Challenges

- If they withdraw further, shift to a less intense topic or check their comfort level.
- If you sense extreme distress, propose relaxation steps or a pause.

Reflection Questions

- Did acknowledging the silence or body language help them disclose more?
- How might you continue using these gentle reflections?

Real life application
Melanie went quiet whenever her father's name came up. The therapist said, "I notice you get very still when we discuss him." Melanie admitted she felt shame over a family conflict, finally opening that door.

Worksheet 29: Eliciting Clarification

Title
Eliciting Clarification

The Purpose
You add a simple question like, "Did I get that right?" after a reflection, letting the client refine your understanding and preventing miscommunication.

The Rationale

Barrett-Lennard (1993) notes that inviting clarification shows respect for the client's perspective. It encourages them to polish your interpretation.

Step-by-Step Instructions

1. Offer a reflection summarising what they said.
2. Follow with, "Is that how you see it, or would you put it differently?"
3. Welcome their correction or elaboration.
4. Incorporate any new details into a refined reflection.

Tips for Debriefing

- Keep your tone curious rather than apologetic.
- Affirm their edits, showing appreciation for helping you understand better.

Troubleshooting Common Challenges

- If they say "yes" automatically, ask a more specific question.
- If they seem unsure how to clarify, offer simpler phrasing for them to confirm.

Reflection Questions

- How does being asked for clarification affect your comfort?
- Does it make you feel more or less heard?

Real life application

A therapist paraphrased Chris's issues, then asked if this was accurate. Chris added another detail they'd missed, and the revised reflection addressed all his concerns more precisely.

Worksheet 30: Reflecting Self-Compassion

Title

Reflecting Self-Compassion

The Purpose
You highlight areas where a client might be overly harsh on themselves, offering a kinder reflection that acknowledges effort and humanity.

The Rationale
Neff (2011) explains that self-compassion fosters personal growth. Reflecting it back helps clients adopt a gentler inner voice.

Step-by-Step Instructions

1. Listen for self-criticism: "I'm a complete mess."
2. Reflect the feeling but add compassion: "It sounds like you're exhausted and blaming yourself, though you've been trying hard despite tough circumstances."
3. Observe how they respond.
4. Encourage them to see the difference between healthy accountability and punishing self-blame.

Tips for Debriefing

- Keep your tone soothing, not patronising.
- Ask how it would feel to treat themselves like a caring friend would.

Troubleshooting Common Challenges

- If they reject kinder language, gently probe why.
- If they're used to tough self-talk, small steps might be needed.

Reflection Questions

- What's the difference between acknowledging mistakes and harshly criticising yourself?
- How might you show yourself more kindness day to day?

Real life application
Bella used to call herself "worthless" for not meeting fitness goals. The therapist reflected, "You're disappointed, but you're also juggling work and childcare. Maybe it's not just you at fault." Bella felt relief, seeing external factors contributed too.

Worksheet 31: Revisiting Past Reflections

Title
Revisiting Past Reflections

The Purpose
You bring up reflections from earlier sessions or moments, seeing if the client's stance has evolved and how fresh insights might emerge.

The Rationale
Norcross and Lambert (2018) suggest continuity in therapy helps clients integrate new realisations. Revisiting older reflections can highlight progress or ongoing blocks.

Step-by-Step Instructions

1. Recall a key reflection from a prior talk: "Last time, we noticed you felt trapped in your job."
2. Ask if that still resonates or if anything changed.
3. Reflect their update: "Now you see a possible exit strategy, which is new."
4. Encourage them to track how their mindset shifts over time.

Tips for Debriefing

- Show genuine interest in their growth.
- Compare older feelings with current ones to celebrate progress or identify areas stuck.

Troubleshooting Common Challenges

- If they forgot the old reflection, recap it briefly.
- If no changes occurred, emphasise it's fine; not all processes are quick.

Reflection Questions

- How have your thoughts shifted since we last explored this?
- Does seeing continuity help you feel more hopeful or aware?

Real life application

A counsellor reminded Mike how he once felt hopeless about finances. Mike now reported feeling more confident after setting a budget plan, showing a marked change since the initial reflection.

Worksheet 32: Reflective Listening in Conflict

Title
Reflective Listening in Conflict

The Purpose
You practise using reflections during tense exchanges or disagreements, validating both sides and reducing antagonism.

The Rationale
Gottman (1999) found that affirming feelings on each side fosters calmer resolutions. Reflecting can cool heated dynamics by showing genuine hearing.

Step-by-Step Instructions

1. Role-play or note a real conflict scenario.
2. Reflect each person's perspective: "You feel disrespected," "They feel unheard."
3. Maintain neutrality, not siding with either viewpoint.
4. Prompt them to notice areas of common ground or shared goals.

Tips for Debriefing

- Stress that you respect everyone's feelings equally.
- Keep your tone calm, even if the parties are agitated.

Troubleshooting Common Challenges

- If conflict escalates, encourage a break or separate reflections.
- If one side insists they're right, gently reflect that stance while leaving room for the other.

Reflection Questions

- Did hearing each side reflected lessen frustration?
- How might each person use this experience to improve communication?

Real life application

During a couple's quarrel, the therapist echoed both partners' grievances without taking sides. Each felt heard, cooling the argument enough to discuss compromises.

Worksheet 33: Complex Trauma Reflections

Title

Complex Trauma Reflections

The Purpose

You refine how you reflect experiences for clients with trauma backgrounds, ensuring gentle, validating language that respects possible triggers.

The Rationale

Herman (1997) emphasises safety and care in trauma work. Reflecting with extra sensitivity prevents re-traumatisation and promotes trust.

Step-by-Step Instructions

1. Use a calm, slow tone; check if they're comfortable before proceeding.
2. Reflect both the content and the emotional weight of a trauma memory: "It sounds like that memory brings intense fear and sadness."
3. Offer immediate support if they become distressed.
4. Confirm they can pause or shift topics any time.

Tips for Debriefing

- Praise the bravery it takes to share.
- Offer grounding techniques or breaks if they feel overwhelmed.

Troubleshooting Common Challenges

- If flashbacks or strong emotional reactions occur, halt in-depth reflection and focus on stability (breathing or grounding).
- If they close off, give them the lead on how far to go.

Reflection Questions

- How did acknowledging your pace and control help you feel safer?
- Which supportive resources might you want to consider next?

Real life application
A client disclosed a past trauma. The therapist repeated it softly, validating the terror and sorrow, then asked if they needed a short grounding exercise. This gentle approach allowed the client to share without feeling flooded.

Worksheet 34: Amplification vs. Undershooting

Title
Amplification vs. Undershooting

The Purpose
You experiment with slightly exaggerating or downplaying the emotion or intensity of a client's statement, inviting them to clarify their real level of feeling.

The Rationale
Miller and Rollnick (2013) say strategic over- or under-reflection can encourage clients to refine or correct. This leads to a more precise understanding of their emotions.

Step-by-Step Instructions

1. Take a statement like, "I'm bothered by my colleague."
2. Reflect in an amplified way: "It sounds like you're absolutely furious?"
3. See if they correct it to "Not furious, just annoyed."
4. Try an undershoot: "You're mildly upset?" and note if they intensify or confirm.

Tips for Debriefing

- Keep an empathetic tone, clarifying you're testing for accuracy.
- Use minimal exaggeration to avoid feeling manipulative.

Troubleshooting Common Challenges

- If they feel mocked, apologise and explain your purpose.
- If no clarification emerges, revert to standard reflections.

Reflection Questions

- Did amplifying or minimising help them find a more exact emotion?
- How might this technique refine your future reflections?

Real life application
Yvonne said she was "kind of stressed" about deadlines. The therapist amplified it: "It's overwhelming you," leading Yvonne to correct, "Well, it's not overwhelming, but it is nagging me daily." This clarified her moderate stress level.

Worksheet 35: Reflecting Motivation Shifts

Title
Reflecting Motivation Shifts

The Purpose
You pay attention when a client's motivation level changes—either up or down—reflecting it so they explore possible causes and solutions.

The Rationale
Prochaska and DiClemente (1983) highlight that readiness fluctuates. Spotting these shifts helps tailor support or strategies promptly.

Step-by-Step Instructions

1. Notice statements indicating a change (e.g., from "I might" to "I'm ready").
2. Reflect the switch: "It seems like you're more determined this week than last."
3. Ask about factors prompting this rise or decline.

4. Discuss what can sustain or restore their drive.

Tips for Debriefing

- Keep curiosity, not judgement: "It's interesting you feel more hopeful now."
- Reinforce any positive jump in motivation as a sign of progress.

Troubleshooting Common Challenges

- If motivation dropped, explore obstacles or discouragement.
- If they can't identify why, help brainstorm possibilities (stress, successes, environment).

Reflection Questions

- Which new event or mindset triggered the shift?
- How can you maintain or boost your current motivation?

Real life application

Theo arrived saying, "I'm not sure about therapy," then ended the session stating, "I want to continue." The therapist noted his stronger tone of commitment, prompting Theo to detail what changed his mind—feeling listened to.

Worksheet 36: Dialectical Reflections

Title

Dialectical Reflections

The Purpose

You hold two contrasting truths at once in a single reflection, teaching the client it's possible to have conflicting feelings or views simultaneously.

The Rationale

Linehan (1993) suggests this approach helps clients accept complexity, rather than forcing a single viewpoint or ignoring conflict.

Step-by-Step Instructions

1. Identify opposing statements (e.g., "I want freedom," "I fear being alone").
2. Reflect both sides: "You crave independence but also worry about loneliness."
3. Encourage them to explore how these can coexist.
4. See if new insights or middle-ground solutions emerge.

Tips for Debriefing

- Validate that life rarely offers all-or-nothing solutions.
- Gently remind them both feelings are valid.

Troubleshooting Common Challenges

- If the client demands an either/or, remind them both feelings can be real.
- If they seem overwhelmed, help them pick small ways to honour each side.

Reflection Questions

- How does accepting both truths affect your choices?
- Which small step respects both sides?

Real life application

Laura felt torn about living alone or staying with her parents. The therapist said, "You want your own space and still yearn for family closeness," letting Laura realise she could find a place nearby, balancing both needs.

Worksheet 37: Prompting Ownership

Title
Prompting Ownership

The Purpose
You reflect the ways clients already take responsibility for their actions, reinforcing they have a role in shaping outcomes.

The Rationale

Ryan and Deci (2000) confirm that realising personal agency fosters motivation. Clients who see their part in change often invest more in the process.

Step-by-Step Instructions

1. Listen for examples of their initiative: "I tried journaling once."
2. Reflect it: "You took a step by experimenting with journaling. That's yours."
3. Ask how it felt to make that effort.
4. Encourage them to see themselves as active agents, not passive recipients.

Tips for Debriefing

- Emphasise self-determination: "This is your journey."
- Congratulate them on each step they initiate.

Troubleshooting Common Challenges

- If they credit others or luck for every positive move, gently point to their personal involvement.
- If they fear blame, clarify you're recognising empowerment, not assigning fault.

Reflection Questions

- Which actions make you feel more in charge of your life?
- How can you expand on that sense of ownership?

Real life application

Naomi said she contacted a career coach on her own. The therapist reflected, "You took that brave step yourself." Naomi felt more confident for deciding her path rather than waiting on circumstances.

Worksheet 38: Appreciative Reflections

Title
Appreciative Reflections

The Purpose
You emphasise small victories and personal strengths in your reflections, helping the client internalise a sense of optimism.

The Rationale
Sheldon and Lyubomirsky (2006) suggest that positive feedback can improve wellbeing. By regularly highlighting positives, you foster an encouraging environment.

Step-by-Step Instructions

1. Notice any accomplishment or effort in the session.
2. Reflect it appreciatively: "You handled that setback with real courage."
3. Allow them to respond or build on the positive recognition.
4. Keep notes of such moments for later reinforcement.

Tips for Debriefing

- Stay specific rather than vaguely complimenting.
- Link the appreciation to concrete examples of their behaviour or qualities.

Troubleshooting Common Challenges

- If they deflect praise, gently ask why they find it hard to accept.
- Avoid overdoing it; keep a balanced approach.

Reflection Questions

- How do you feel hearing specific appreciation?
- Which accomplishment do you value most?

Real life application
Jerome felt unsure about therapy progress. The therapist reflected, "You attended every session this month, showing consistency and commitment." Jerome's self-doubt eased, seeing that consistency as evidence of caring about his well-being.

Worksheet 39: Reflecting Goals and Progress

Title
Reflecting Goals and Progress

The Purpose
You tie the client's current challenges back to their main objectives, highlighting how each small step—or setback—relates to the bigger journey.

The Rationale
Miller and Rollnick (2013) emphasise that drawing lines between daily hurdles and ultimate aims keeps motivation alive, reminding them why each step counts.

Step-by-Step Instructions

1. Recall the client's stated goal: "You aim to be more confident socially."
2. Show how current struggles connect: "This anxiety you felt at the party is part of learning to handle social situations."
3. Reflect any progress or insights.
4. Encourage them to see the broader perspective.

Tips for Debriefing

- Acknowledge even partial improvements.
- Summaries can spark new ways to overcome current barriers.

Troubleshooting Common Challenges

- If they lose sight of goals, restate them clearly, reinforcing original motivations.
- If stuck, break goals into smaller tasks so progress feels attainable.

Reflection Questions

- Did linking this issue to your main goal help you stay committed?
- What next step fits into your bigger plan?

Real life application
Sasha wanted better public speaking skills. The therapist reflected how volunteering

for a small work presentation aligned with that aim, framing it as a practical move forward.

Worksheet 40: Inviting Reassessment

Title
Inviting Reassessment

The Purpose
You conclude each session by reflecting main themes, then prompting the client to re-evaluate their current feelings or commitments, ensuring ongoing clarity.

The Rationale
Miller and Rollnick (2013) advise regular check-ins about how the session influenced motivation. This can solidify next steps or reveal new concerns.

Step-by-Step Instructions

1. Summarise the key points or emotions expressed.
2. Ask: "How do you feel about your goals or approach now?"
3. Reflect any changes or stable stances they mention.
4. Plan what to address or try before the next session.

Tips for Debriefing

- Encourage honesty about doubts or new ideas.
- Use open questions that let them express fresh perspectives.

Troubleshooting Common Challenges

- If they seem unsure, rephrase or offer a simple scale-based question.
- If time is short, keep this step brief yet purposeful.

Reflection Questions

- Which part of today's discussion stands out most for you?

- Are you leaving with clarity or new questions?

Real life application

Brian ended a session by reviewing his breakthroughs. Asked how he felt now, he said more committed to daily journaling. This simple check-in reinforced his readiness before leaving.

By honing these 40 reflective listening exercises, you enhance the dialogue's depth and support clients in understanding themselves. Thoughtful reflections transform everyday exchanges into powerful moments of clarity and growth.

Rolling with Resistance

This category shows how to handle pushback or reluctance in a non-confrontational way. Worksheets guide you to validate the client's feelings and gently explore underlying worries. By 'rolling with' instead of fighting against resistance, you preserve rapport and find more productive pathways for growth.

Worksheet 1: Resistance Cues

Title
Resistance Cues

Purpose
You learn to spot verbal or nonverbal signals of resistance early, preparing gentle and understanding responses that encourage open dialogue.

The Rationale
Miller and Rollnick (2013) note that recognising subtle signs of resistance allows therapists to adapt their approach swiftly. By addressing client hesitancy with empathy rather than force, you transform potential standoffs into collaborative moments.

Step-by-Step Instructions

1. Create two columns on a sheet: **Observed Cue** and **Potential Response**.
2. In "Observed Cue," list examples (folded arms, abrupt changes of topic, sighs, refusal to discuss a matter).
3. In "Potential Response," plan a reflective or validating statement.
4. Review which cues are most frequent in your sessions and refine your planned responses over time.

Tips for Debriefing

- Stress that these cues aren't stubbornness but signals of discomfort or fear.
- Encourage the client to correct you if your response isn't helpful.

Troubleshooting Common Challenges

- If you miss a cue, don't panic. Note it for future sessions.
- If the client remains closed off, reflect the possibility they feel uneasy or pressured.

Reflection Questions

- Which cue do you notice most often in your sessions?
- How does planning gentle responses change your approach?

Real life application

Marina noticed her client typically crossed arms and looked away when overwhelmed. She prepared an empathetic statement—"You seem uneasy about this topic"—leading the client to acknowledge stress and talk more freely.

Worksheet 2: Shifting the Client's Perspective

Title
Shifting the Client's Perspective

Purpose
You learn to step into the client's stance instead of debating them. This defuses defensiveness by affirming they have reasons for their views.

The Rationale
Miller and Rollnick (2013) explain that aligning with the client's viewpoint before offering new perspectives can reduce pushback. Validating their logic fosters trust and openness to alternate ideas.

Step-by-Step Instructions

1. Listen to the client's objections or fears.
2. Reflect them accurately: "It sounds like you really doubt if this plan can help."
3. Affirm what's sensible in their stance: "Given past disappointments, that makes sense."
4. Gently introduce a new angle without dismissing their concerns.

Tips for Debriefing

- Highlight that their doubts are normal, not wrong.
- Give them time to respond or correct your summary.

Troubleshooting Common Challenges

- If they remain fixed, maintain a collaborative tone.
- If you sense tension easing, carefully suggest exploring an alternative approach.

Reflection Questions

- How does validating their stance first affect their willingness to hear other ideas?
- Which common objections might you be more open to now?

Real life application

Robert insisted therapy wouldn't help. The therapist agreed, "It's logical you'd be sceptical after past attempts." Realising he was heard, Robert relaxed enough to consider smaller next steps.

Worksheet 3: Validation Exercises

Title
Validation Exercises

Purpose
You practise offering genuine validation of a client's feelings or experiences, which often softens defences and promotes a sense of safety.

The Rationale
Rogers (1957) emphasises that clients need authentic acceptance. Validating them helps lower resistance because they feel less judged and more open to collaboration.

Step-by-Step Instructions

1. Listen for emotional statements ("I'm so angry," "I'm overwhelmed").
2. Provide a validation that acknowledges their reality: "It's understandable you'd feel that way given…."
3. Write down examples of validation phrases.
4. Check the client's response to see if they seem relieved or calmer.

Tips for Debriefing

- Validation is not agreement but understanding; clarify that you respect their emotion's legitimacy.

- Keep your tone warm, without minimising what they're going through.

Troubleshooting Common Challenges

- If the client doubts your sincerity, keep it brief and specific.
- If they reject validation, respond gently, "Your feelings are yours, and it's okay to have them."

Reflection Questions

- Which type of validation statement felt most natural for you?
- How did validating their emotion shift the conversation?

Real life application

Lauren, exasperated about her job, heard, "It makes sense to be frustrated after working so hard without recognition." Feeling seen, she opened up further about her resentments.

Worksheet 4: Exploring the 'No'

Title

Exploring the 'No'

Purpose

You discover what truly drives a client's refusal, diving beneath the surface to uncover hidden worries, values, or misunderstandings.

The Rationale

According to Miller and Rollnick (2013), every "no" holds valuable clues. By respectfully examining it, you address the real barrier instead of pushing in vain.

Step-by-Step Instructions

1. When the client says "no" to an idea, pause and reflect: "It seems you're not open to that right now."
2. Ask, "Could you share what's behind that feeling?"

3. Listen for deeper reasons—fear of failure, lack of resources, contradictory goals.
4. Discuss how these insights might guide a more suitable approach.

Tips for Debriefing

- Emphasise you're not forcing them to comply but seeking understanding.
- Show that "no" doesn't end the conversation but begins exploration.

Troubleshooting Common Challenges

- If they refuse to elaborate, respect their boundary and revisit later.
- If they reveal a misunderstanding, clarify gently.

Reflection Questions

- Did learning the reason behind "no" shift your perspective on how to help?
- How might you adapt the plan to fit their concerns?

Real life application
Anna rejected the idea of group therapy. Probing further, the therapist learned Anna feared judgment from peers. They decided on one-on-one sessions first, easing Anna into the concept of group support later.

Worksheet 5: Reflecting Resistance

Title
Reflecting Resistance

Purpose
You reflect the client's resistant statements directly, letting them hear their own reluctance echoed back neutrally, which may prompt self-inquiry or revision.

The Rationale
Miller and Rollnick (2013) teach that simply re-stating a resistant comment can lead

the client to clarify or soften. Resistance is less likely to escalate if met with calm reflection.

Step-by-Step Instructions

1. Identify a resistant statement: "I don't want to try that."
2. Reflect it without judgment: "You really feel that approach isn't for you right now."
3. Wait for them to respond, perhaps explaining further.
4. Maintain empathy throughout, avoiding confrontation.

Tips for Debriefing

- Keep your tone steady, showing you hear them fully.
- If they expand on their resistance, reflect that new detail too.

Troubleshooting Common Challenges

- If they ramp up defensiveness, stay composed and mirror their stance: "This is clearly frustrating for you."
- If they quickly apologise or retract, assure them their initial reaction was valid.

Reflection Questions

- Did repeating their words spark any shift in their tone or reasoning?
- How did this reflection technique differ from trying to persuade them otherwise?

Real life application

Cole stated, "Talking about my family is pointless." The therapist calmly repeated, "You believe discussing your family won't help." Cole then elaborated on past unhelpful experiences, revealing deeper trust issues.

Worksheet 6: Use of Paradox

Title
Use of Paradox

Purpose
You occasionally agree with the client's reluctance in a seemingly paradoxical way, prompting them to argue for the opposite side. This technique must be used gently.

The Rationale
Miller and Rollnick (2013) highlight paradoxical statements as a strategic tool. When you appear to accept their inertia, clients may instinctively defend the possibility of change.

Step-by-Step Instructions

1. Sense a stalemate or strong resistance (e.g., "I'll never quit smoking").
2. Offer a paradoxical reflection: "You're so set that quitting might never happen—maybe continuing to smoke is your best choice now."
3. Observe if they rebut, saying "Well, maybe I can quit eventually."
4. Handle their new stance with care, guiding them to articulate what might make quitting possible.

Tips for Debriefing

- Ensure your tone is calm, not sarcastic.
- If the client becomes offended, revert to standard validation.

Troubleshooting Common Challenges

- Avoid overusing paradox, as it can feel manipulative.
- If they take your statement literally, clarify you were mirroring their stance to explore deeper motivations.

Reflection Questions

- Did paradox spur any surprising shift?
- How can you use it sparingly yet effectively?

Real life application
Amy insisted she'd never lose weight. The therapist responded, "Maybe staying the

same is the best option for now." Surprised, Amy confessed she did want to try smaller changes, opening the door to practical steps.

Worksheet 7: Emotional Regulation for Practitioners

Title
Emotional Regulation for Practitioners

Purpose
You note your own internal reactions to a client's resistance, developing techniques to remain calm and empathetic rather than defensive.

The Rationale
Hill (2010) stresses that a therapist's emotional self-awareness can prevent conflict escalation. If you stay centred, you model calmness.

Step-by-Step Instructions

1. After a session, reflect on moments you felt frustrated or triggered.
2. Name the emotion and why it arose (e.g., fear of failure, personal triggers).
3. Develop coping strategies (deep breathing, grounding, mental affirmations).
4. Practise these techniques when you sense tension building.

Tips for Debriefing

- Remind yourself the client's resistance often reflects their internal struggles, not personal rejection.
- Seek peer support or supervision if a certain style of resistance repeatedly affects you.

Troubleshooting Common Challenges

- If your stress is high, consider short breaks or transitional exercises in session.
- If you react strongly, briefly apologise and refocus on the client's feelings.

Reflection Questions

- What triggered your reaction?
- Which calming method helps you stay compassionate?

Real life application

Thomas felt slighted when a client dismissed all his suggestions. Realising frustration, he paused to breathe and silently reminded himself that the client's reluctance stemmed from fear, not personal attack.

Worksheet 8: Brainstorming Small Shifts

Title

Brainstorming Small Shifts

Purpose

You explore minor, manageable changes rather than large leaps, preventing overwhelm or rebellion if the client finds big steps too daunting.

The Rationale

According to Prochaska and DiClemente (1983), taking tiny steps can reduce resistance. Clients often accept micro-adjustments more readily than radical transformations.

Step-by-Step Instructions

1. Ask, "What's one tiny modification you could consider right now, if any?"
2. List multiple micro-options: adjusting a routine by five minutes, trying a new coping skill once.
3. Check their comfort level for each suggestion.
4. Help them pick one to test, emphasising no pressure to do more until ready.

Tips for Debriefing

- Celebrate the client's choice of even a small step.
- Reassure them they can pause or scale back if it still feels too big.

Troubleshooting Common Challenges

- If they reject all suggestions, reflect that it's okay to wait until they find one that fits.
- If they overshoot, remind them the point is to avoid feeling swamped.

Reflection Questions

- Which micro-step feels truly achievable this week?
- How might a small success motivate larger changes?

Real life application
Shane refused to overhaul his diet. Instead, they agreed he'd add a piece of fruit each morning. Achieving that small goal gave Shane confidence, paving the way for more significant nutritional improvements later.

Worksheet 9: Reflective Curiosity

Title
Reflective Curiosity

Purpose
You practise a stance of genuine curiosity—asking neutral questions that invite clients to explore their reluctance or doubt without feeling pushed.

The Rationale
Hill (2010) advocates open inquiry that's free of judgment. Curiosity fosters openness and can uncover overlooked solutions or motivations.

Step-by-Step Instructions

1. Notice a resistant statement, e.g., "I can't see this helping."
2. Respond with curiosity: "What leads you to feel it won't help?"
3. Reflect or paraphrase their explanation, still maintaining interest: "So it seems past attempts left you discouraged?"
4. Follow up if they hint at deeper reasons.

Tips for Debriefing

- Keep your tone warm, not interrogative.
- Affirm that you value their perspective even if you see things differently.

Troubleshooting Common Challenges

- If they clam up, try a simpler question or reframe.
- If they lash out, mirror their frustration calmly, acknowledging the difficulty of the topic.

Reflection Questions

- Did approaching them with curiosity help them share more?
- How might you bring this mindset to other tense moments?

Real life application
A client repeatedly said, "I'm not the type for therapy." The therapist asked, "What about it do you think won't fit you?" This led the client to reveal fears about judgment, allowing reassurance and new rapport.

Worksheet 10: No Pressure Agreement

Title
No Pressure Agreement

Purpose
You assure the client that they can move at their own pace. Eliminating perceived coercion often reduces resistance and preserves dignity.

The Rationale
Deci and Ryan (2008) emphasise that autonomy fosters genuine engagement. Letting clients know they control timing and choices can lower defensive barriers.

Step-by-Step Instructions

1. Acknowledge the client's concerns about feeling pushed.
2. State explicitly: "You're free to choose how fast or slow you go here."

3. Reflect any relief or residual tension they exhibit.
4. Explore smaller steps only if they feel ready.

Tips for Debriefing

- Reassure that you'll still support them regardless of how they proceed.
- Mention that refusal now doesn't mean it's forever off the table.

Troubleshooting Common Challenges

- If they test your sincerity, remain calm and reaffirm their autonomy.
- If they want you to decide everything, gently guide them back to their own authority.

Reflection Questions

- Did feeling free to say no reduce your defensiveness?
- Which area do you still feel unsure about?

Real life application
Nico resisted any plan, fearing pressure. The therapist clearly stated he could decide if or when to try new strategies. Feeling respected, Nico later volunteered to test a single coping skill.

Worksheet 11: Collaborative Re-Framing

Title
Collaborative Re-Framing

Purpose
You and the client jointly reshape how they see a problem, aligning it more with their perspective and reducing feelings of being misunderstood.

The Rationale
Miller and Rollnick (2013) highlight that co-creating reframes ensures the client feels valued. This increases ownership and lowers friction.

Step-by-Step Instructions

1. Ask, "How do you view this issue, in your own words?"
2. Offer a preliminary reframe: "Could it be that…?"
3. Invite them to refine or correct your version.
4. Finalise a reframe that resonates with them, preserving their voice in the process.

Tips for Debriefing

- Emphasise that you want their input to capture the problem realistically.
- Show appreciation if they correct you—that means you're learning together.

Troubleshooting Common Challenges

- If they disagree entirely, revert to their own phrasing or viewpoint.
- If they feel pressured to adopt your wording, reassure them this is a mutual effort.

Reflection Questions

- How does re-framing together shift your sense of control over the problem?
- Did the new viewpoint feel more accurate?

Real life application
A teen disliked the label "defiant." The therapist suggested co-creating a different phrase: "You're protective of your independence." The teen liked it, feeling this described his situation more fairly.

Worksheet 12: Pacing Your Responses

Title
Pacing Your Responses

Purpose

You practise waiting a moment before replying to resistant remarks. This breathing space often cools tension and lets the client reflect.

The Rationale

Hill (2010) notes that pausing fosters emotional regulation for both parties. It prevents impulsive retorts, allowing calmer, empathic reflections.

Step-by-Step Instructions

1. When the client resists or shows frustration, pause for a few seconds.
2. Observe your own reaction, exhale slowly if needed.
3. Offer a measured reflection: "You're not feeling comfortable with this idea."
4. See if the client's stance shifts with the calmer energy.

Tips for Debriefing

- If pausing feels awkward, remember it's brief and purposeful.
- A small silence can prompt the client to rephrase or explain further.

Troubleshooting Common Challenges

- If the client rushes you, maintain composure and then respond gently.
- If they fill the silence with more resistance, reflect that new statement.

Reflection Questions

- Did waiting enhance clarity or empathy in your response?
- How might pacing shape future interactions?

Real life application

Sarah felt combative about changing her schedule. The therapist took a short breath before reflecting, "It's tough to consider altering your routine right now." This calm approach reduced Sarah's irritation.

Worksheet 13: Supportive Pause

Title
Supportive Pause

Purpose
You intentionally pause mid-session for a short reflective break, signalling acceptance and allowing the client to gather thoughts without feeling rushed.

The Rationale
Rogers (1957) saw value in gentle pauses. They reassure clients they're not pressed to produce answers quickly and can lower agitation.

Step-by-Step Instructions

1. Notice moments when tension is high or confusion arises.
2. Announce a short pause: "Let's take a moment to breathe."
3. Sit quietly for ten or twenty seconds.
4. Ask if anything new emerged in that silence.

Tips for Debriefing

- The client might share fresh insights or decide they want to revisit a point.
- If they dislike silence, invite them to use it for calm reflection rather than forced quiet.

Troubleshooting Common Challenges

- If they feel awkward, keep the pause short and supportive.
- If they keep talking, honour their preference for continuous speech.

Reflection Questions

- Did the pause help you see your thoughts more clearly?
- Would you like to use these mini-breaks more often?

Real life application
Martin became anxious discussing finances. The therapist suggested a brief pause. After a few silent breaths, Martin admitted he was afraid of appearing irresponsible, leading to a more honest conversation about budgeting fears.

Worksheet 14: Seeking Permission

Title
Seeking Permission

Purpose
You ask the client if they're open to hearing suggestions or information, reinforcing their autonomy and reducing pushback.

The Rationale
Deci and Ryan (2008) show that granting clients choice fosters intrinsic motivation. Asking, "May I offer an idea?" respects their freedom and often lowers defensiveness.

Step-by-Step Instructions

1. Recognise a moment where you might share a thought or advice.
2. Say, "Is it okay if I share a perspective?" or "May I offer a suggestion?"
3. If they decline, respect that. If they agree, offer your idea briefly.
4. Ask for feedback on whether it resonates.

Tips for Debriefing

- Emphasise they can say "no" without repercussions.
- Keep suggestions short and open-ended, so they can adapt them if needed.

Troubleshooting Common Challenges

- If they often refuse, remain supportive and wait for their readiness.
- If they look uneasy, reaffirm their right to pass on your input.

Reflection Questions

- Did inviting them to accept or decline your idea build trust?
- How can you use permission checks more frequently?

Real life application

Maria was hesitant about new coping strategies. The therapist asked, "Would you like to hear a simple technique others found helpful?" Maria appreciated the courtesy, felt in control, and agreed to listen.

Worksheet 15: Normalize Skepticism

Title
Normalize Skepticism

Purpose
You frame a client's sceptical attitude as understandable, reducing any shame or frustration they might feel for doubting the process.

The Rationale
Miller and Rollnick (2013) explain that clients who sense acceptance of their doubts are more likely to stay engaged. Normalising scepticism shows you respect their caution.

Step-by-Step Instructions

1. When they express doubt, acknowledge it: "It's very normal to feel unsure."
2. Reflect: "Many people have had the same hesitations."
3. Encourage them to explore where that doubt comes from.
4. Clarify that caution can be part of a healthy decision-making process.

Tips for Debriefing

- Emphasise that you've seen others move forward despite initial scepticism.
- Remind them that their pace is valid.

Troubleshooting Common Challenges

- If they interpret normalising as dismissing, gently clarify you accept the seriousness of their concerns.

- If they remain stuck, invite them to share more about their experiences with past solutions.

Reflection Questions

- How does hearing your doubt is common affect your perception?
- Does it feel more comfortable discussing your reservations now?

Real life application
Kevin repeatedly voiced scepticism about therapy. The therapist responded, "It's common to question if this really helps, especially if you've tried before. We can see together if this approach might fit better." Kevin felt less defensive, opening further discussion.

Worksheet 16: Revisiting Goals

Title
Revisiting Goals

Purpose
You circle back to the client's self-stated goals when they resist certain approaches, gently reminding them why these aims matter to them.

The Rationale
Prochaska and DiClemente (1983) found that reconnecting a current hurdle with personal aspirations can reignite motivation. Highlighting their original reasons for seeking help can ease tension.

Step-by-Step Instructions

1. Note the moment the client resists a suggestion.
2. Calmly recall the goal they set: "You mentioned you wanted to feel less anxious at night…"
3. Ask if that goal remains meaningful.
4. Suggest how a proposed step might align with that goal, leaving space for their input.

Tips for Debriefing

- Do not use the goal to shame them, but to guide them back to their own priorities.
- If they changed goals, confirm the new direction is valid.

Troubleshooting Common Challenges

- If they feel pressured, stress that they can adjust the goal or method.
- If they forgot their earlier aim, recap it gently.

Reflection Questions

- Did reconnecting with your original aspiration shift your stance?
- Which part of your goal still feels most inspiring?

Real life application
Selena resisted tracking her mood. The therapist recalled how Selena wanted better sleep and calmer evenings, linking mood tracking to spotting sleep disruptors. Selena realised the alignment and agreed to try for a week.

Worksheet 17: Resistance Journal

Title
Resistance Journal

Purpose
You encourage the client to log moments of resistance—what they felt, thought, or did—between sessions, to discuss and dissect them later.

The Rationale
Miller and Rollnick (2013) propose journaling about resistance can transform it from an emotional reaction into a reflective exercise. It clarifies triggers and patterns.

Step-by-Step Instructions

1. Give them a simple template with columns: **Situation**, **Resistant Thought**, **Emotional State**, **Outcome**.
2. Ask them to fill it whenever they notice themselves pushing back on an idea or suggestion.
3. In the next session, review entries to identify common themes.
4. Brainstorm how to handle those triggers differently.

Tips for Debriefing

- Stress there's no judgment—resistance is normal data to explore.
- Praise any honest entries, even if it's just one or two.

Troubleshooting Common Challenges

- If they forget or find it tedious, suggest short bullet points.
- If they worry about revealing negative feelings, reassure them it's a helpful exploration.

Reflection Questions

- Did journaling highlight any patterns or triggers you hadn't seen before?
- How might you respond differently next time?

Real life application
Jake recorded times he resisted changing his exercise routine. He noticed a pattern: he always balked when tired after work, realising a morning routine might face less pushback.

Worksheet 18: Gauging Motivation Dip

Title
Gauging Motivation Dip

Purpose
You check if the client feels their drive declining, investigating reasons behind the slump and gently addressing them before resistance deepens.

The Rationale

Prochaska and DiClemente (1983) emphasise that motivation isn't constant. Detecting early dips can prevent total disengagement.

Step-by-Step Instructions

1. Periodically ask: "Are you feeling less motivated about this lately?"
2. Invite them to rate their current motivation compared to before.
3. Discuss factors behind any dip (e.g., stress, doubts, time constraints).
4. Brainstorm how to reignite or adjust the plan so it stays feasible.

Tips for Debriefing

- Be calm; a dip doesn't mean failure.
- Emphasise it's normal and can be addressed with small modifications.

Troubleshooting Common Challenges

- If they feel ashamed, normalise that everyone's motivation ebbs and flows.
- If they can't identify a cause, you can offer possible triggers or reassess goals.

Reflection Questions

- Which external or internal factors brought motivation down?
- How might you tweak your routine or approach to restore enthusiasm?

Real life application

Mia admitted feeling a drop in her resolve to reduce sugar intake. She and the therapist realised new work stress was draining her. Adding a stress-management step helped her regain some momentum.

Worksheet 19: Humor in Defusing Tension

Title

Humor in Defusing Tension

Purpose
You consider how gentle, respectful humour can ease a tense moment of resistance, showing empathy and shared humanity without trivialising the client's concern.

The Rationale
Seligman (2011) suggests that mild humour often lightens mood, bridging gaps. If done carefully, it can break defensiveness by reminding the client you're both human.

Step-by-Step Instructions

1. When tension spikes, gauge if a minor humorous remark might fit (e.g., "That's a totally normal reaction—I'd probably be rolling my eyes too if I were you!").
2. Check the client's body language to ensure they're not offended.
3. If they smile or relax, continue. If not, revert to a more serious tone.
4. Reflect on whether humour helped them open up.

Tips for Debriefing

- Keep humour light and self-deprecating if needed, never mocking them.
- Stop if the client shows discomfort or annoyance.

Troubleshooting Common Challenges

- If they have a painful topic, humour may be inappropriate.
- If you sense forced laughter, ease back and offer empathy instead.

Reflection Questions

- Did the lightness help you feel more relaxed or accepted?
- How might humour be used sparingly to support tough discussions?

Real life application
Rita got tense talking about budgeting. The therapist made a small quip about "We accountants at heart" in a playful tone. Rita grinned, tension eased, and they resumed discussing finances more calmly.

Worksheet 20: Empathy Retrieval

Title
Empathy Retrieval

Purpose
When resistance spikes, you pause to reaffirm your empathy, letting the client see you're an ally rather than an opponent.

The Rationale
Rogers (1957) posits that re-rooting in empathy during conflict can quell resistance, reminding clients you're there to understand, not dictate.

Step-by-Step Instructions

1. If a session grows tense, pause.
2. Restate your desire to grasp their feelings: "I really want to see this from your side."
3. Ask if they can help clarify what's hardest in this moment.
4. Reflect or paraphrase with extra care, showing you respect their viewpoint.

Tips for Debriefing

- Keep your voice calm and gentle, emphasising genuine care.
- Mention that you value their honesty, even if it's frustration directed at you.

Troubleshooting Common Challenges

- If they refuse further discussion, honour their boundary, offering to revisit later.
- If you sense strong emotion, stay consistent in your empathic approach rather than switching to solutions.

Reflection Questions

- How did reminding them of your empathy affect the atmosphere?
- Did they open up any new angles?

Real life application
Jasmine lashed out, feeling misunderstood. The therapist softly said, "I genuinely want to feel what this is like from your perspective. Help me get it right." Jasmine calmed and explained her struggle more fully.

Worksheet 21: Conscious Choice Focus

Title
Conscious Choice Focus

Purpose
You highlight the client's right to make decisions, framing actions as a conscious choice rather than something forced upon them, which reduces defensive reactivity.

The Rationale
Deci and Ryan (2008) note that emphasising autonomy fosters lasting commitment. When they see every step as their choice, they're less likely to resist.

Step-by-Step Instructions

1. Notice if they feel forced: "It sounds like you think you 'have to' do this."
2. Reassure: "It's truly up to you how to proceed."
3. Reflect how each option has pros and cons, but remains their call.
4. Encourage them to consider which choice aligns with their goals.

Tips for Debriefing

- Keep a neutral stance, not subtly pushing a direction.
- Validate the burden of deciding while supporting their self-determination.

Troubleshooting Common Challenges

- If they want you to decide for them, gently remind them that their ownership matters.
- If they mention external pressures, explore how to handle those while retaining personal agency.

Reflection Questions

- How does knowing it's your decision influence your sense of control?
- Which path feels most aligned with your values?

Real life application

After repeated discussions, Sam said he felt pressured to attend group therapy. The therapist emphasised it's his choice, listing possible positives but affirming he could refuse. Feeling his autonomy respected, Sam eventually decided to give group therapy a try.

Worksheet 22: Scaling Resistance

Title

Scaling Resistance

Purpose

You treat resistance as a numeric value, turning it into a problem-solving task. This helps you and the client target specific factors that might reduce tension.

The Rationale

Rollnick and Allison (2004) propose rating scales to clarify issues. Clients identifying a "resistance score" often become curious about how to lower it, fostering collaborative brainstorming.

Step-by-Step Instructions

1. Ask, "On a scale of 1–10, how resistant do you feel to exploring this change?"
2. Let them define the number.
3. Ask, "What might shift it down by even one point?"
4. Discuss small, actionable ideas and measure progress over time.

Tips for Debriefing

- Remind them a single-point shift is valuable.
- Validate any reason behind their chosen number.

Troubleshooting Common Challenges

- If they refuse to rate, explore a simpler approach (mild, moderate, strong resistance).
- If they rate it extremely high, check if smaller goals or a different approach might help.

Reflection Questions

- Which factor keeps your resistance at that number?
- How might you reduce it a notch?

Real life application

Julie rated her resistance to journaling at 8. Searching for ways to drop it to a 7, she realised a lighter schedule (just a few lines nightly) felt less burdensome, letting her test it without feeling overwhelmed.

Worksheet 23: Learning from Past Attempts

Title

Learning from Past Attempts

Purpose

You explore times the client tried to change but encountered strong pushback or gave up, extracting valuable lessons that might reduce current resistance.

The Rationale

Bandura (1997) suggests revisiting past efforts can clarify what worked or failed. This helps avoid repeating unhelpful approaches and builds on prior successes.

Step-by-Step Instructions

1. Prompt, "When have you tried something like this before?"

2. Reflect on how resistance played a role then—was it from themselves, others, or external factors?
3. Discuss what they learned or could do differently now.
4. Note any small successes or near-successes to replicate.

Tips for Debriefing

- Encourage them to see "failures" as a trial that offered insights.
- Focus on problem-solving, not blaming themselves or the process.

Troubleshooting Common Challenges

- If they become discouraged remembering old failures, reframe them as experiences.
- If they blame external reasons, reflect how they might adapt within those constraints.

Reflection Questions

- Which past stumbling block can you avoid or handle differently?
- Did you discover any hidden strengths in your older attempts?

Real life application
Ryan tried to quit smoking three times, each time feeling pressured by family. Now he realises the external push triggered defiance. They planned a self-driven strategy this time, hopefully reducing internal resistance.

Worksheet 24: Check for Misinformation

Title
Check for Misinformation

Purpose
You clarify if the client's resistance stems from incorrect beliefs or assumptions about a method, offering gentle facts to correct misunderstandings.

The Rationale
Rollnick and Miller (1995) say that misperceptions can fuel undue resistance. Providing accurate info in a respectful way can soften reluctance.

Step-by-Step Instructions

1. If the client states a questionable belief, reflect it calmly: "You've heard that therapy only works if you're 'crazy.'"
2. Ask if it's okay to share a different perspective or evidence.
3. Gently provide correct info, e.g., "Therapy often supports everyday stress, not just severe disorders."
4. See if their stance shifts or if they need more time to consider.

Tips for Debriefing

- Avoid a lecturing tone.
- Encourage them to think critically about the new info rather than just accept or reject it.

Troubleshooting Common Challenges

- If they cling to the misinformation, remain kind, acknowledging it takes time to shift beliefs.
- If they feel patronised, reaffirm their autonomy to accept or explore data.

Reflection Questions

- How does having clearer information change your perspective?
- Are there any other doubts you want to address?

Real life application
Kara resisted using medication, believing it created addiction in all cases. The therapist gently explained how certain prescriptions are safe short-term, with doctor oversight. Kara softened her stance, requesting more info from a trusted physician.

Worksheet 25: Mirror the Ambivalence

Title
Mirror the Ambivalence

Purpose
You offer a double-sided reflection that captures both the client's reasons to continue and their reasons to change, acknowledging internal conflict without pushing either side.

The Rationale
Miller and Rollnick (2013) highlight double-sided reflections as a method to integrate conflicting feelings, reducing tension and clarifying possible directions.

Step-by-Step Instructions

1. Listen for statements showing conflicting attitudes: "I want to eat healthier, but I love junk food."
2. Reflect both sides: "On one hand, you value better nutrition; on the other, you enjoy the comfort of junk food."
3. Ask which side feels stronger or more urgent right now.
4. Explore how to address the tension.

Tips for Debriefing

- Keep your reflection neutral, not pushing one side.
- Validate it's normal to hold two opposing views.

Troubleshooting Common Challenges

- If they see this as contradictory, gently reassure it's common to want two things at once.
- If they feel stuck, suggest discussing possible small experiments that honour both sides.

Reflection Questions

- Did hearing both sides out loud help you recognise any pattern?
- Which factor do you want to prioritise today?

Real life application

Briana, torn about leaving her job, heard the therapist reflect, "You cherish the stability yet long for a role that challenges you more." She admitted her biggest fear was risk, but also a strong desire for growth. Recognising both drove her to research new roles carefully.

Worksheet 26: Trigger Analysis

Title

Trigger Analysis

Purpose

You identify events, words, or settings that activate a client's resistance, creating a plan to reduce or handle these triggers more effectively.

The Rationale

Skinner (1953) suggests that behaviour often arises in response to specific cues. Mapping triggers can reduce unconscious pushback and support smoother progress.

Step-by-Step Instructions

1. Ask the client to recall times they felt sudden defiance or reluctance.
2. Note what happened right before (a phrase you used, a memory, a certain environment).
3. Brainstorm ways to avoid or reshape each trigger.
4. Encourage them to notice and log triggers in real life.

Tips for Debriefing

- Remind them triggers can be emotional or external events.
- Develop alternative reactions or "safe words" if they feel triggered in session.

Troubleshooting Common Challenges

- If triggers are complex or deep-rooted, consider small steps first.
- If they feel embarrassed about certain triggers, maintain an accepting stance.

Reflection Questions

- Which triggers are most common for you?
- What small adjustment could decrease that trigger's intensity?

Real life application

Karen always resisted talk about childhood. Realising the word "family" triggered her, the therapist agreed to use gentler phrasing like "early home life," so Karen felt less defensive discussing it.

Worksheet 27: Recalibrating the Plan

Title
Recalibrating the Plan

Purpose
You and the client step back to adjust the overall approach if resistance consistently remains high, focusing on more attainable changes or a slower timeline.

The Rationale
Prochaska and DiClemente (1983) caution that pushing clients too far beyond readiness raises opposition. Recalibrating keeps them engaged and hopeful.

Step-by-Step Instructions

1. Acknowledge persistent resistance: "It seems we're stuck with the current plan."
2. Ask if they'd prefer different goals, smaller tasks, or more flexible pacing.
3. Rewrite the action steps, emphasising feasibility.
4. Check how they feel about this revised approach.

Tips for Debriefing

- Affirm that recalibration isn't quitting; it's adapting to real circumstances.
- Compare the new plan with their main goals to ensure alignment.

Troubleshooting Common Challenges

- If they see recalibration as failure, reframe it as a wise modification.
- If they oversimplify the plan, confirm it still challenges them slightly.

Reflection Questions

- Does the updated plan feel more realistic?
- Which change are you now willing to try?

Real life application
Colin hated logging food daily, stalling all progress. They agreed to track just one meal a day, feeling less burdened. This small shift made him more consistent with the project.

Worksheet 28: Revisiting Emotional Safety

Title
Revisiting Emotional Safety

Purpose
You assess whether the client feels safe sharing doubts or frustrations. If trust is low, you reinforce a non-judgemental environment before pushing further changes.

The Rationale
Rogers (1957) stresses that a sense of safety is crucial for honest disclosure. Without it, clients often resist to protect themselves.

Step-by-Step Instructions

1. Mid-session, ask if they feel safe discussing their reservations: "Is there anything making you feel uneasy or judged?"
2. Reflect any concerns they voice: "You worry I'll push you too fast."
3. Reassure them they lead the pace.
4. Confirm again that all feelings—even reluctance—are welcome.

Tips for Debriefing

- Affirm their right to stop or change direction if they feel unsafe.
- Adjust topics or techniques if they show signs of discomfort.

Troubleshooting Common Challenges

- If they refuse to discuss safety, remain patient and leave the door open for the future.
- If they name a specific fear, brainstorm ways to address it promptly.

Reflection Questions

- Does feeling safe make it easier to explore tough topics?
- How might you tell me if you feel unsafe again?

Real life application
Lily was edgy each time therapy got personal. On asking about safety, she admitted fear of being criticised. The therapist assured her of unconditional respect, and Lily relaxed, willing to explore deeper.

Worksheet 29: Finding Shared Understanding

Title
Finding Shared Understanding

Purpose
You search for any overlap between the client's stance and yours—common values or goals—to re-establish a collaborative foundation.

The Rationale
Miller and Rollnick (2013) emphasise that identifying shared ground reduces an "us vs. them" dynamic. Clients see you as an ally rather than an adversary.

Step-by-Step Instructions

1. Listen for mutual interests: improved well-being, less stress, improved relationships.
2. Reflect the commonality: "We both want you to feel happier at work."
3. Ask how you can build on this shared wish.
4. Use it as a reference point whenever conflict arises.

Tips for Debriefing

- Keep references to mutual goals succinct and direct.
- Validate that differences remain, but a key overlap can unite your efforts.

Troubleshooting Common Challenges

- If they claim no common ground, consider a broader perspective or smaller sub-goals.
- If they accept the shared point, gently revolve solutions around it.

Reflection Questions

- Which area do we clearly agree on?
- How can that agreement guide our steps forward?

Real life application
Stan disliked the idea of budgeting. But both he and the therapist agreed his main goal was reducing financial stress for family stability. Highlighting this objective helped him stay open to trying small financial changes.

Worksheet 30: Reflect and Redirect

Title
Reflect and Redirect

Purpose
You respond to resistance by mirroring the resistant statement, then gently shifting focus to a more constructive angle, allowing a new perspective to emerge.

The Rationale

Miller and Rollnick (2013) show that tension decreases when you first accept the client's statement, then invite them to consider alternate approaches.

Step-by-Step Instructions

1. Hear the resistant claim: "Therapy is just talking; it can't fix real problems."
2. Reflect: "So you feel therapy might not solve the real issues."
3. Redirect: "Could we look at smaller pieces of the problem therapy might help with?"
4. Observe if they entertain exploring partial help.

Tips for Debriefing

- Keep your redirect subtle, not dismissive of their worry.
- Applaud their willingness to try any piece that feels manageable.

Troubleshooting Common Challenges

- If they stay stuck, accept that for now and show readiness to revisit later.
- If they pivot, follow them into discussing small steps or areas they might tolerate exploring.

Reflection Questions

- Which part of your problem do you think we could tackle first?
- Did blending reflection with a gentle new path feel less confrontational?

Real life application

Claudia insisted that talking wouldn't fix her job issues. The therapist repeated this stance, then suggested starting with smaller stressors at work that therapy could address, prompting cautious agreement.

Worksheet 31: Socratic Questioning

Title
Socratic Questioning

Purpose
You use open-ended questions to help the client examine their own reasons for resistance, prompting self-discovery rather than direct persuasion.

The Rationale
Beck (2011) states that guided questioning lets clients uncover assumptions or biases. They become more receptive upon seeing their own thought patterns.

Step-by-Step Instructions

1. Focus on a resistant statement: "I just can't handle another failure."
2. Pose curious questions: "What do you think would happen if you did try? How do you see failure?"
3. Let them reflect or correct misconceptions.
4. Follow up: "What could it look like if it partially succeeded?"

Tips for Debriefing

- Use a calm, inquisitive tone, not interrogation.
- Summarise their insights to confirm clarity.

Troubleshooting Common Challenges

- If they say "I don't know," offer time to think or rephrase.
- If they get defensive, affirm their feelings and try gentler questions.

Reflection Questions

- Did exploring your own reasons reveal anything new?
- Which question shifted your understanding the most?

Real life application
Dana was rigidly opposed to diet changes. The therapist asked, "What's your biggest worry about trying a new way?" and "If it partly worked, how would life be different?" Dana realised fear of total failure overshadowed the possibility of partial gains.

Worksheet 32: Encourage Self-Validation

Title
Encourage Self-Validation

Purpose
You guide the client to articulate the pros of their caution or reluctance, evaluating if it truly helps them or stands in the way, shifting them from auto-resistance to a thoughtful stance.

The Rationale
Rogers (1957) suggests that letting clients affirm their own caution fosters deeper reflection. When they hear themselves describe each reason, they can judge its utility more objectively.

Step-by-Step Instructions

1. Ask them to list reasons they believe resistance is good or protective.
2. Reflect each reason, ensuring you show acceptance.
3. Prompt them to consider if these reasons still serve their long-term goals.
4. Gently inquire, "What do you want to do next, knowing these reasons?"

Tips for Debriefing

- Affirm that caution can be wise, not just a barrier.
- Empathise with any fear of being rushed or judged.

Troubleshooting Common Challenges

- If they strongly defend each reason, reflect that they find comfort in not changing.
- If they spot a reason that's outdated, encourage them to see it as progress to let it go.

Reflection Questions

- Which reason for caution still feels valid?
- Which reason might be holding you back more than helping?

Real life application

Jay had multiple rationales for resisting therapy. He listed how it protected him from disappointment. Then realising it also isolated him, he decided some caution was needed, but not to the point of avoidance.

Worksheet 33: Addressing Fear of Failure

Title

Addressing Fear of Failure

Purpose

You recognise that reluctance often ties to a fear of trying and not succeeding. By validating this fear, you help clients see mistakes as learning opportunities rather than proof of inability.

The Rationale

Bandura (1997) underscores that fear of failure can breed avoidance. Normalising slip-ups encourages perseverance instead of quitting at the first stumble.

Step-by-Step Instructions

1. Acknowledge their fear: "You worry about failing again."
2. Reflect times they succeeded at smaller tasks.
3. Discuss how failure can offer lessons, not just shame.
4. Suggest micro-goals to reduce the perceived risk of an all-or-nothing outcome.

Tips for Debriefing

- Show empathy for disappointment in past attempts.
- Reinforce that many success stories come after initial setbacks.

Troubleshooting Common Challenges

- If they remain paralysed by fear, propose experiments with minimal risk.
- If they reference previous humiliations, gently reflect that trauma while framing new tries as different contexts.

Reflection Questions

- What's your worst-case scenario if you try?
- Could partial success still bring some benefits?

Real life application
Lucy resisted applying for jobs after repeated rejections. The therapist acknowledged her fear and pointed out she once found a good fit after months of searching. This boosted her courage to update her CV and try again.

Worksheet 34: Drawing on Past Adaptability

Title
Drawing on Past Adaptability

Purpose
You help the client recall times they adapted to new situations successfully, countering the belief they cannot handle further changes.

The Rationale
Egan (2013) states that recounting past adaptability fosters self-belief. Realising they overcame challenges before reduces current resistance.

Step-by-Step Instructions

1. Prompt them: "Tell me about a time you adapted to a major change."
2. Reflect the strengths they used—creativity, patience, resourcefulness.
3. Invite them to compare that situation to now, asking, "Could those strengths help here?"
4. See if recalling past flexibility lessens today's hesitation.

Tips for Debriefing

- Focus on highlighting effort, not luck, to strengthen their sense of capability.
- Avoid glossing over tough feelings; normalise that change can be stressful but still manageable.

Troubleshooting Common Challenges

- If they claim they've never adapted well, gently suggest smaller examples.
- If they remain sceptical, reiterate any partial successes you recall or see.

Reflection Questions

- Which quality from that past success do you still have?
- How can you apply it to this current challenge?

Real life application
After losing a job before, Paul once learned new skills. He'd forgotten that victory. Recalling how he adapted to tech changes at work, he felt more confident facing another uncertain work transition.

Worksheet 35: Joint Problem-Solving

Title
Joint Problem-Solving

Purpose
You transform a moment of resistance into collaborative brainstorming, emphasising that you value the client's input and want to find solutions together.

The Rationale
Miller and Rollnick (2013) affirm that clients often resist if they feel dictated to. Partnering on ideas fosters investment and creativity.

Step-by-Step Instructions

1. When they resist a suggestion, respond: "Let's figure something out together."

2. Ask them for a proposal or adjustment: "What might you change in that idea to make it acceptable?"
3. Gather multiple options, letting them lead or co-lead.
4. Pick a plan they feel comfortable testing.

Tips for Debriefing

- Affirm that their perspective matters more than any generic method.
- Keep your role as a guide, not an authority imposing rules.

Troubleshooting Common Challenges

- If they say "I don't know," gently prompt small ideas or partial steps.
- If they propose unrealistic strategies, reflect potential pitfalls, still praising their initiative.

Reflection Questions

- Did collaborating reduce tension?
- Which proposed solution feels most promising?

Real life application

Lena refused to track her spending. The therapist asked how she'd like to approach budgeting differently. Lena offered a weekly "check-in" method with phone reminders. Her ownership increased cooperation.

Worksheet 36: Break Tasks into Micro-Steps

Title
Break Tasks into Micro-Steps

Purpose
You chunk a large goal into tiny actions when the client resists or feels overwhelmed. Each small task is more palatable, decreasing refusal.

The Rationale

Prochaska and DiClemente (1983) show incremental successes build confidence. Clients less frequently reject micro-steps, seeing them as doable.

Step-by-Step Instructions

1. Identify a big task they resist.
2. Split it into micro-pieces (e.g., gather supplies, set a five-minute timer to begin, record a short note).
3. Confirm which micro-step feels feasible.
4. Encourage them to celebrate each micro-win.

Tips for Debriefing

- Keep instructions super-clear, so the step is unmistakable and easy to complete.
- Emphasise that mastering small tasks can lead to bigger changes later.

Troubleshooting Common Challenges

- If they still hesitate, break it down further.
- If the step is too small to matter, ensure it aligns with a bigger chain of progress.

Reflection Questions

- Which micro-step are you comfortable trying now?
- How might completing that mini-task increase your confidence?

Real life application

Grant refused a daily mindfulness practice. They scaled it down to a single minute of focusing on breath each morning. Successfully doing that small action made Grant more open to a two-minute routine next week.

Worksheet 37: Empower the Client as Expert

Title
Empower the Client as Expert

Purpose
You invite the client to propose strategies themselves, positioning them as the authority on their life. This bypasses the feeling of being lectured.

The Rationale
Deci and Ryan (2008) stress autonomy. By honouring the client's own ideas, they're more likely to accept or refine them rather than resist.

Step-by-Step Instructions

1. State clearly: "You know your situation best. How might you address this challenge?"
2. Let them brainstorm potential actions.
3. Reflect each idea, exploring feasibility.
4. If needed, gently offer suggestions only after hearing theirs.

Tips for Debriefing

- Applaud creative or out-of-the-box thoughts.
- If they draw a blank, encourage small or even silly ideas to spark creativity.

Troubleshooting Common Challenges

- If they say "I have no ideas," propose a brainstorming prompt or recall past solutions they tried.
- If their proposals are extreme, reflect possible pros and cons without dismissing them outright.

Reflection Questions

- Which idea feels most exciting or realistic?
- How does taking the lead boost your motivation?

Real life application
Tori repeatedly refused the therapist's coping strategies for panic. Asked for her own

ideas, Tori devised a short mental "safe place" visualisation. She felt ownership and was willing to practise it.

Worksheet 38: Reflecting Potential Regret

Title
Reflecting Potential Regret

Purpose
You sensitively reflect how staying with the current behaviour might lead to future regret, inviting the client to weigh consequences without feeling scolded.

The Rationale
Miller and Rollnick (2013) show that gently highlighting possible long-term downsides can nudge contemplation. This reflection must be free of blame to remain effective.

Step-by-Step Instructions

1. Note the client's expressed desire for a different outcome.
2. Reflect softly: "If this pattern continues, you might look back wishing you'd tried something else."
3. Pause for their reaction—do they agree, add detail, or reject the idea?
4. Affirm it's their decision, but you sense they'd hate to miss out on their goal.

Tips for Debriefing

- Keep your tone empathic, not ominous or guilt-inducing.
- Emphasise it's about caring for future well-being.

Troubleshooting Common Challenges

- If they get defensive, revert to summarising their current feelings.
- If they say they don't care about future consequences, validate that stance and explore immediate benefits or costs.

Reflection Questions

- How might you feel in a year if you remain on this path?
- Does considering future regret shift anything for you now?

Real life application

Kara resisted saving money. The therapist gently said, "One day, you may regret not building some security. Does that ring true?" Kara admitted she feared ending up financially dependent on others, becoming more open to a budget plan.

Worksheet 39: Summarizing Progress

Title

Summarizing Progress

Purpose

Even if a session feels tough, you highlight small forward steps or insights, ensuring a positive note that may lower residual resistance.

The Rationale

Rogers (1957) states that noticing any progress helps keep clients engaged. Wrapping up with a recap shows them they moved forward despite challenges.

Step-by-Step Instructions

1. Near session's end, list any achievements—clarifications, a shift in perspective, or small agreement.
2. Reflect the effort they put in: "You hung in there even while doubting."
3. Reinforce how these small gains align with their bigger aims.
4. Ask how they feel, heading out with that awareness.

Tips for Debriefing

- Maintain sincerity; avoid inflating trivial changes.
- Invite the client to add or correct any progress points you missed.

Troubleshooting Common Challenges

- If they insist no progress happened, gently highlight even minor steps or new information.
- If the session was very conflict-ridden, find at least one neutral or positive takeaway.

Reflection Questions

- Which tiny success or fresh insight stands out for you?
- How can you build on it between now and next time?

Real life application
Felix felt the session was futile. The therapist reminded him he'd clarified why he resists quitting vaping. Realising that self-awareness was indeed a step, Felix left feeling less defeated.

Worksheet 40: Ending on a Respectful Note

Title
Ending on a Respectful Note

Purpose
You conclude by reinforcing respect for the client's feelings and choices, showing readiness to continue whenever they're prepared, leaving minimal tension.

The Rationale
Miller and Rollnick (2013) affirm that finishing on a note of mutual respect preserves the therapeutic relationship. Clients feel safe to return and re-engage.

Step-by-Step Instructions

1. Summarise the main points of the session, especially areas of resistance or progress.
2. Say something like, "I appreciate your honesty today. This is your journey, and I'm here to support however you decide."
3. Thank them for sharing, even if it included resistance.
4. Invite them to revisit or shift directions next time, emphasising it's all valid.

Tips for Debriefing

- Keep a calm tone and steady eye contact if suitable.
- Reassure them they can change their mind or refine their goals later.

Troubleshooting Common Challenges

- If they remain upset, gently ask if they want a brief plan for coping until next session.
- If they're still uncertain, honour that uncertainty as part of their process.

Reflection Questions

- How does ending on respect make you feel about coming back?
- Are there any final concerns you'd like to address next time?

Real life application

Tom was grumpy about the session, saying he felt no improvement. The therapist thanked him for being candid and reminded him that the pace is his choice. Tom left with less animosity, agreeing to keep the next appointment.

Developing Discrepancy

These worksheets help highlight the gap between a client's current behaviours and their larger goals or values. By gently revealing inconsistencies, you spark reflection that can prompt change. This method encourages clients to see for themselves why new choices might serve their deeper ideals.

Worksheet 1: Value Sorting

Title
Value Sorting

Purpose
You help clients clarify what they hold dear by arranging values in order of importance. This reveals where current behaviours might clash with these top-priority principles.

The Rationale
Miller and Rollnick (2013) suggest that developing discrepancy often starts by highlighting how actions veer from personal ideals. Sorting core values can make the gap more visible, motivating clients to realign.

Step-by-Step Instructions

1. Provide a list or deck of value cards (family, integrity, career success, health, etc.).
2. Ask the client to rank them from most to least significant.
3. Encourage them to reflect briefly on each chosen priority.
4. Explore if any daily habit contradicts the top values and note any reflections.

Tips for Debriefing

- Ask open questions about how they feel seeing certain values at the bottom of the list.
- Emphasise there are no "wrong" values; it's about personal truth.

Troubleshooting Common Challenges

- If they're overwhelmed by too many values, pick a shorter list or let them group similar ones.
- If they resist ranking, encourage approximate groupings (very important, somewhat important, less important).

Reflection Questions

- Which high-ranking value did you rarely think about before?
- Does any recent behaviour work against your top values?

Real life application
Sandra sorted her values, realising "creative expression" mattered more than she thought. Recognising her long work hours left no room for art, she felt uneasy, seeing how she neglected something vital to her sense of self.

Worksheet 2: Where Am I Now vs. Where I Want to Be

Title
Where Am I Now vs. Where I Want to Be

Purpose
You guide clients to describe their current situation and their ideal future, spotlighting the gap that can inspire helpful shifts.

The Rationale
According to Prochaska and DiClemente (1983), examining a future vision next to present reality clarifies discrepancies, fuelling desire to act.

Step-by-Step Instructions

1. Ask the client to sketch or write about how things stand now (health, relationships, finances).
2. Then have them describe how they'd prefer each area in an ideal scenario.
3. Compare the two versions side by side.
4. Discuss the differences that catch their attention most.

Tips for Debriefing

- Encourage honesty, including positives in the present so it's balanced.
- Emphasise that no one's path is linear—this is about noticing, not judging.

Troubleshooting Common Challenges

- If the client struggles imagining an ideal future, suggest small improvements rather than grand transformations.
- If they feel discouraged, normalise that acknowledging gaps can be hard but also empowering.

Reflection Questions

- Which specific area shows the biggest gap?
- How do you feel seeing these differences?

Real life application
Max wrote about his current daily routine (feeling lethargic, unmotivated) and contrasted it with his wish to be energetic and engaged in hobbies. Spotting the contrast pushed him to consider small daily changes.

Worksheet 3: Cost-Benefit Worksheet

Title
Cost-Benefit Worksheet

Purpose
You and the client identify short- and long-term gains and downsides of both maintaining the status quo and embracing change, creating a clear contradiction in priorities.

The Rationale
Miller and Rollnick (2013) describe cost-benefit analysis as a powerful method for revealing how short-term comforts can lead to long-term harm, nudging clients toward healthier choices.

Step-by-Step Instructions

1. Divide a page into two columns: **Staying the Same** and **Making the Change**.
2. Under each, list short-term benefits, short-term costs, long-term benefits, and long-term costs.
3. Examine each quadrant carefully, ensuring details are specific.

4. Compare and see if the long-term gains of change outweigh the short-term comforts of doing nothing.

Tips for Debriefing

- Let the client define each benefit or cost; avoid substituting your view.
- If they feel stuck, ask about daily frustrations or hopes.

Troubleshooting Common Challenges

- If they highlight many negatives for change, reflect understanding but gently probe potential overlooked positives.
- If it triggers strong guilt or shame, remind them it's normal to weigh pros and cons carefully.

Reflection Questions

- Which column surprised you?
- Does anything stand out as an immediate call to action?

Real life application
Aaron saw that staying up late felt good short-term (entertainment, no bedtime routine), but the long-term cost was poor health and missed morning productivity. Acknowledging this, he became more open to a better sleep schedule.

Worksheet 4: Behaviour-Value Map

Title
Behaviour-Value Map

Purpose
You help clients draw connections between specific behaviours and their central values, revealing how each habit either supports or undermines what matters most to them.

The Rationale

Miller and Rollnick (2013) highlight the impact of visual mapping in developing discrepancy. Seeing lines from behaviour to value can be a wake-up call that fosters reflection.

Step-by-Step Instructions

1. List key values on one side (family, honesty, self-care).
2. List regular behaviours on another side (smoking, skipping exercise, volunteering).
3. Draw arrows indicating whether each behaviour supports or contradicts a value.
4. Discuss which contradictions feel most pressing to address.

Tips for Debriefing

- Keep it simple at first. Too many items can overwhelm.
- If they see few direct links, help them consider broader impacts of each behaviour.

Troubleshooting Common Challenges

- If they avoid acknowledging contradictions, gently offer examples: "How does skipping family gatherings mesh with your strong family value?"
- If they see multiple contradictions, let them pick one to focus on for now.

Reflection Questions

- Which behaviour-value link hits you hardest?
- How do you feel about behaviours that undermine your top value?

Real life application

Liz mapped her nightly TV bingeing to her value of career progress. She realised the time drained her focus for study. Recognising this gap made her cut back on screen time, devoting an hour to professional training instead.

Worksheet 5: Role Exploration

Title
Role Exploration

Purpose
You have the client examine the different roles they fill (e.g., parent, friend, employee) and check for alignment or conflict in how they live those roles.

The Rationale
Egan (2013) notes that when someone's behaviour clashes with role expectations or personal identity in that role, tension arises. Examining roles clarifies those friction points.

Step-by-Step Instructions

1. List each role: "Worker," "Parent," "Spouse," "Volunteer," etc.
2. Under each, have them describe ideal traits or responsibilities.
3. Compare those ideals with current habits.
4. Circle any glaring mismatches and reflect on how that feels.

Tips for Debriefing

- Validate that it's normal for roles to clash sometimes.
- Encourage them to see small improvements in each role rather than feeling they must perfect them all at once.

Troubleshooting Common Challenges

- If they find too many demands, remind them that recognising conflicts is the first step to prioritising.
- If guilt arises, emphasise self-compassion and incremental changes.

Reflection Questions

- Which role do you feel proudest of? Why?
- Which role do you think needs more attention?

Real life application
Martin saw he wanted to be a supportive father, yet he spent all evenings working.

Realising how that clashed, he arranged more family time, starting with reading bedtime stories regularly.

Worksheet 6: Personal Inventory Check

Title
Personal Inventory Check

Purpose
You and the client create a snapshot of daily activities or habits, rating how each fits their life mission or highest goals, identifying possible contradictions.

The Rationale
Prochaska and DiClemente (1983) suggest that a daily habit inventory can highlight patterns the client might overlook. Any mismatch stands out, prompting deeper thought.

Step-by-Step Instructions

1. Have the client list out routine tasks or habits (morning coffee, commute, workout, social media scrolling).
2. Next to each, rate from 0–10 how well it aligns with a key life goal.
3. Observe which habits have low scores.
4. Explore strategies to adjust or replace those low-score habits if desired.

Tips for Debriefing

- Keep the list manageable—maybe 5–10 daily habits.
- Affirm that it's normal to have some low-score items; you're not condemning them, just noticing.

Troubleshooting Common Challenges

- If they dismiss the idea that these small habits matter, gently ask how it all adds up across days or weeks.
- If they see many habits scored low, prioritise one or two to tackle first.

Reflection Questions

- Which daily habit's score most surprised you?
- How might you improve or reduce that habit to better fit your goals?

Real life application
Dina rated her late-night phone scrolling a 2/10 for her "quality sleep" goal. This realisation prompted her to set a "no devices after 10 p.m." rule, slowly improving her rest.

Worksheet 7: Future Impact Visualization

Title
Future Impact Visualization

Purpose
You help the client imagine how current behaviour might shape their relationships or dreams long-term, revealing consequences they may not have considered.

The Rationale
Bandura (1997) affirms that visualising future outcomes can spark motivation to adjust present choices. Making it vivid deepens emotional resonance.

Step-by-Step Instructions

1. Ask the client to close their eyes (or write) and picture themselves 5 or 10 years from now if they continue current habits.
2. Prompt them to note feelings, environment, and relationships in this scenario.
3. Reflect any discrepancies with what they want for themselves.
4. Encourage them to describe how a small change today might alter that future image.

Tips for Debriefing

- Reinforce that the future isn't fixed; they can shape it.

- If the vision is bleak, handle emotional distress by offering empathy and focusing on potential solutions.

Troubleshooting Common Challenges

- If they struggle to visualise, ask smaller increments or a specific domain (career or health).
- If it triggers anxiety, reassure them it's a thought exercise to guide empowerment.

Reflection Questions

- What stood out in your future vision?
- What small step could shift that future in a more positive direction?

Real life application
Nick pictured himself in 10 years, still in unhealthy relationships and exhausted at work, missing out on family life. This stark vision motivated him to seek therapy to manage stress and improve communication skills.

Worksheet 8: Highlighting Competing Interests

Title
Highlighting Competing Interests

Purpose
You help the client place two conflicting desires side by side—like wanting financial stability but loving impulsive spending—so they can see the conflict clearly.

The Rationale
Miller and Rollnick (2013) emphasise that identifying contradictory yearnings can push clients to choose or strike a healthier balance, rather than drifting in ambivalence.

Step-by-Step Instructions

1. Ask about each desire: "What do you like about spontaneous spending? What do you like about saving money?"
2. Write them in two columns.
3. Reflect back the tension: "Both appear important to you, yet they clash."
4. Prompt the client to brainstorm ways to honour both or prioritise one.

Tips for Debriefing

- Avoid judgment about which side is "better."
- Encourage them to see if certain compromises might exist.

Troubleshooting Common Challenges

- If they cling to both extremes, normalise that conflict and see if partial solutions can emerge.
- If they claim a solution is impossible, gently ask about any small steps or middle ground.

Reflection Questions

- Which side feels stronger or more urgent today?
- Could you give each side a fair share in your life?

Real life application

Alma valued travel but also dreamt of owning a home. Through listing both sets of interests, she decided to allocate a fixed percentage for travel and the rest for a home savings plan, honouring both sides somewhat.

Worksheet 9: Letter to a Mentor

Title
Letter to a Mentor

Purpose
You encourage the client to write an imaginary letter to someone they respect,

explaining their current struggle in aligning values with behaviours. This externalises the discrepancy, often clarifying it.

The Rationale

Egan (2013) suggests letter-writing as a creative method to clarify internal conflicts. Addressing a respected figure can reduce defensiveness and enhance sincerity.

Step-by-Step Instructions

1. Have them pick a mentor or admired person (real or fictional).
2. Write a letter describing how they feel stuck and why their actions don't match their ideals.
3. Ask them to reflect on what the mentor might reply.
4. Encourage them to share any insights gleaned from the exercise.

Tips for Debriefing

- Let them keep the letter private or read excerpts if they wish.
- Praise their willingness to explore vulnerability in this imaginative format.

Troubleshooting Common Challenges

- If they can't think of a mentor, they can address it to an older version of themselves or a wise character.
- If the letter brings sadness or shame, offer empathy and reassurance that this is about growth, not guilt.

Reflection Questions

- What did writing to someone you admire reveal about your true aims?
- Did imagining their response help you see solutions?

Real life application

Tony wrote to his beloved grandmother, who championed honesty and kindness. The process reminded him how much he treasured those values but felt he was slipping by gossiping at work. He decided to watch his language to honour her memory.

Worksheet 10: Mirroring Contradictions

Title
Mirroring Contradictions

Purpose
You reflect back contradictory statements a client makes, gently highlighting how they're holding two conflicting positions. This invites them to reconcile or choose a direction.

The Rationale
Miller and Rollnick (2013) indicate that hearing one's own contradictory statements fosters self-exploration and potential resolution. This technique must be free of blame.

Step-by-Step Instructions

1. Note contradictory remarks (e.g., "I want to lose weight" and "I hate cooking, so I always grab fast food").
2. Reflect both in one statement: "You really want a healthier body, yet you avoid cooking entirely."
3. See if the client corrects or explores the contradiction.
4. Ask, "How do you think both can exist at once?"

Tips for Debriefing

- Keep the tone gentle; you're not calling them hypocritical, just noticing.
- Acknowledge that ambivalence is common and normal.

Troubleshooting Common Challenges

- If they become defensive, empathise with the difficulty of balancing two strong desires.
- If they brush it off, politely revisit it later as needed.

Reflection Questions

- Which side of the contradiction feels more compelling to you now?
- What small step might unify or lean towards one side?

Real life application
Zara said she yearned for a stable relationship but consistently avoided calls from potential partners. The therapist mirrored this dual stance, prompting Zara to admit a fear of intimacy. She then decided to address that fear in small ways.

Worksheet 11: Goal-Behaviour Gap Analysis

Title
Goal-Behaviour Gap Analysis

Purpose
You list the client's goals and examine each daily action, labelling which ones support or impede each goal, forging a clear picture of mismatched efforts.

The Rationale
Prochaska and DiClemente (1983) found that systematic gap analysis fosters realisation that many daily steps deviate from overarching aims, spurring motivation to change small details.

Step-by-Step Instructions

1. List each primary goal in a column.
2. Under each goal, note relevant daily actions. For each action, mark it as "Supporting," "Neutral," or "Undermining."
3. Spot patterns (e.g., an action that undermines multiple goals).
4. Brainstorm alternatives or modifications to reduce undermining habits.

Tips for Debriefing

- Offer a short list of example actions if they struggle to identify how each habit relates to each goal.
- Celebrate even small supportive actions that might have gone unnoticed.

Troubleshooting Common Challenges

- If they see mostly undermining items, reassure them that noticing is the first step to progress.
- If they feel overwhelmed, pick one goal to focus on at a time.

Reflection Questions

- Which habits negatively affect more than one goal?
- What is the simplest way to adjust or replace those habits?

Real life application

Connor used a table with columns for "Financial Stability" and "Better Physical Health," realising ordering take-out nightly undermined both. This spotlighted meal planning as a way to support finances and health simultaneously.

Worksheet 12: Consequences Timeline

Title

Consequences Timeline

Purpose

You explore potential future outcomes if clients keep their current behaviour, mapping a timeline of likely consequences that might intensify over the years.

The Rationale

Bandura (1997) notes that imagining progressive negative outcomes can break present-minded complacency. A timeline makes the escalation of consequences tangible.

Step-by-Step Instructions

1. Draw a horizontal line, marking increments of 1 or 2 years.
2. Discuss how the same habit, if unchanged, could play out over time.
3. Write possible outcomes (personal, professional, relational) under each time marker.
4. Prompt the client to reflect on which future point most concerns them.

Tips for Debriefing

- Provide empathy if they feel anxious about seeing a bleak potential future.
- Also discuss how positive changes could alter that timeline for balance.

Troubleshooting Common Challenges

- If the client claims they can't predict the future, remind them this is hypothetical, based on current patterns.
- If they become overwhelmed, explore partial solutions or resource-building strategies.

Reflection Questions

- Which future marker is most alarming or motivating for you?
- How might you prevent or lessen these negative projections?

Real life application
Elaine examined her heavy smoking over a 5-year timeline, seeing possible health declines, financial strain, and guilt. Recognising how swiftly issues could worsen, she became more open to a step-by-step quitting approach.

Worksheet 13: Questioning the Status Quo

Title
Questioning the Status Quo

Purpose
You formulate open-ended queries that invite the client to challenge their own routines or assumptions, rather than passively accept them.

The Rationale
Egan (2013) points out that gently questioning "why keep doing this?" can spark introspection. Clients re-examine habits they previously saw as normal.

Step-by-Step Instructions

1. Prepare a series of open-ended prompts: "What keeps you continuing this pattern?" "What might happen if you tried a different approach?"
2. Have the client respond in writing or conversation, taking time to reflect.
3. Summarise key realisations.
4. Ask how they feel about these new insights.

Tips for Debriefing

- Keep the tone curious, never accusatory.
- If they can't answer, let them think further or answer gradually over sessions.

Troubleshooting Common Challenges

- If they become defensive, reaffirm it's about exploring possibilities, not attacking them.
- If they find the question pointless, try rephrasing or linking it directly to a known concern of theirs.

Reflection Questions

- Which question challenged you the most?
- Did any new perspective emerge about your routine?

Real life application
Loren had always used late-night gaming as stress relief. Asked, "What might happen if you replaced an hour of gaming with reading or a calming activity?" he realised he'd likely feel more rested, prompting small changes to his nightly routine.

Worksheet 14: Journaling on Conflict

Title
Journaling on Conflict

Purpose
The client keeps a short journal capturing moments of internal friction—times they sense a mismatch between actions and deeper values—and the emotions felt.

The Rationale

Miller and Rollnick (2013) highlight journaling for self-awareness. Writing about real-time conflicts can underscore how often the client confronts incongruence.

Step-by-Step Instructions

1. Provide a simple format: Date, Situation, Action Taken, Felt Conflict, Emotional Reaction.
2. Ask them to record episodes when they feel they acted against their own principles.
3. Review entries to locate patterns or triggers.
4. Brainstorm ways to reduce or handle those inner clashes.

Tips for Debriefing

- Acknowledge the vulnerability in documenting conflicts.
- Keep the journaling brief so it doesn't feel burdensome.

Troubleshooting Common Challenges

- If they forget, encourage setting a daily alarm to quickly jot down notes.
- If they become ashamed reading entries, offer reassurance that this is a normal growth process.

Reflection Questions

- Which repeated conflict did you see in your journal?
- How might you act differently next time to lessen that discomfort?

Real life application

Kelly noticed multiple times she laughed at jokes she found mean-spirited, feeling guilty afterwards. Recognising this pattern, she resolved to gently speak up or remain quiet instead of giving the impression she agreed.

Worksheet 15: Benefits of Realignment

Title
Benefits of Realignment

Purpose
You lead clients to list specific emotional, relational, or practical advantages they might gain if their actions matched their values more closely.

The Rationale
Miller and Rollnick (2013) emphasise that seeing positive outcomes of bridging the gap can fuel hope. Focusing on gains, not just losses, can break inertia.

Step-by-Step Instructions

1. Ask them to identify ways life could improve by living more in line with core principles.
2. Encourage detail: "Better self-esteem," "Stronger family bonds," "Less regret."
3. Reflect each stated benefit: "That sounds meaningful."
4. Summarise the list to underscore its impact.

Tips for Debriefing

- If they struggle to find positives, gently prompt them about potential relief or pride.
- Affirm that these benefits might not be immediate but still worthwhile.

Troubleshooting Common Challenges

- If they fixate on losses or effort needed, acknowledge those but pivot back to the benefits.
- If they downplay the positives, ask how others might notice or appreciate the change.

Reflection Questions

- Which benefit feels most motivating right now?
- How would your daily life look if you experienced these positives?

Real life application
Emma saw that stopping her weekend binge drinking could mean fewer Monday

headaches, improved work performance, and deeper friendships not centred on partying. These benefits motivated her to reduce drinking outings.

Worksheet 16: Examine Core Beliefs

Title
Examine Core Beliefs

Purpose
You invite the client to explore deep-seated thoughts that might keep them stuck in behaviour-value conflict. Recognising these beliefs can open the door to change.

The Rationale
Beck (2011) argues that core beliefs heavily influence repeated actions. Identifying unhelpful assumptions reveals the roots of discrepancy.

Step-by-Step Instructions

1. Ask about beliefs behind the mismatch: "Why do you think you continue this behaviour despite feeling it's wrong?"
2. Look for statements like, "I'm not capable of better," or "I deserve punishment."
3. Reflect them compassionately, emphasising they're learned beliefs, not truths.
4. Discuss how altering or challenging these beliefs might foster alignment.

Tips for Debriefing

- Show empathy if they uncover painful or entrenched ideas.
- Refer them to deeper cognitive restructuring resources if needed.

Troubleshooting Common Challenges

- If they're reluctant to face these beliefs, normalise that it can feel scary.
- If they blame external forces, reflect that external stress is real yet beliefs can still shape responses.

Reflection Questions

- Which core belief stands out as most influential?
- Is there evidence that counters this belief?

Real life application

Luke believed "I'm worthless unless I'm perfect." This belief led him to sabotage good opportunities from fear of failing. Realising how it contradicted his desire for achievement, he began exploring kinder self-talk.

Worksheet 17: Reflecting on Role Models

Title

Reflecting on Role Models

Purpose

You encourage the client to think of someone they admire who embodies the values or lifestyle they yearn for, revealing the discrepancy between their actions and the life they respect.

The Rationale

Lockwood et al. (2005) highlight that role models can trigger self-reflection. Comparing personal behaviour to admired traits can spark a drive to close that gap.

Step-by-Step Instructions

1. Ask the client to pick a role model—someone living authentically or consistently with principles.
2. Explore which traits or actions they admire.
3. Compare with the client's own behaviour in similar contexts.
4. Brainstorm small steps that emulate those admired qualities.

Tips for Debriefing

- Be mindful if envy arises; reframe it as inspiration.

- If they can't think of a personal contact, famous figures or fictional characters are fine.

Troubleshooting Common Challenges

- If they label themselves "not good enough," remind them role models aren't perfect and invite small approximations.
- If their idol is unrealistic or extreme, focus on specific positive traits they can adapt reasonably.

Reflection Questions

- Which characteristic do you most want to adopt?
- How could you practise that quality in a small, real way?

Real life application
Monica admired her sister's positivity and willingness to admit mistakes. Realising she was defensive when in error, Monica practised saying, "I messed up. Here's how I'll fix it," improving relationships at work.

Worksheet 18: Scaling Discomfort

Title
Scaling Discomfort

Purpose
You gauge how uncomfortable the client feels about their behaviour-value mismatch on a scale from 1–10, sparking discussion on what might intensify or ease that discomfort.

The Rationale
Rollnick and Allison (2004) assert that numeric scales help quantify intangible feelings. Discussing a slight move up or down can yield problem-solving.

Step-by-Step Instructions

1. Identify a behaviour that contradicts a core value.
2. Ask, "How uncomfortable does this conflict make you, from 1–10?"
3. Explore what would shift that discomfort by one or two points.
4. Plan small adjustments that might reduce the mismatch or the stress around it.

Tips for Debriefing

- Encourage honesty in selecting a number—no right or wrong.
- If the discomfort is high, reassure them it shows they deeply care about aligning with values.

Troubleshooting Common Challenges

- If they score low, reflect that maybe they're at peace with the mismatch.
- If they can't think of changes, help them brainstorm or pick an easier scenario to scale first.

Reflection Questions

- Why did you pick that number?
- How could you move it one point higher (or lower)?

Real life application
Candice felt her weekly partying conflicted with wanting to be a dependable mum, rating the discomfort an 8/10. She identified limiting partying to one monthly event could drop that to a 5, making her feel more in line with motherhood values.

Worksheet 19: Root Cause Analysis

Title
Root Cause Analysis

Purpose
You guide the client to delve deeper into emotional or life factors sustaining their behavioural-value discrepancy, unearthing underlying motivations or traumas.

The Rationale

Egan (2013) emphasises that superficial solutions don't last if deeper drivers remain hidden. A root cause discussion can reveal what truly keeps them stuck.

Step-by-Step Instructions

1. Pick a frequent mismatch.
2. Ask "Why do you think this persists?" repeatedly, each time digging further (similar to "5 Whys" technique).
3. Reflect possible emotional ties (fear of judgement, longing for acceptance, unresolved pain).
4. Consider how addressing this root might reduce the conflict at surface level.

Tips for Debriefing

- Stay compassionate; going deep can stir painful memories or vulnerabilities.
- Validate that discovering hidden motives is an important milestone, not an instant fix.

Troubleshooting Common Challenges

- If they get overwhelmed, slow the pace or suggest breaks.
- If they can't find a root cause, normalise that it might reveal itself over time.

Reflection Questions

- Did uncovering these deeper layers make sense of your actions?
- How do you feel about possibly addressing that root?

Real life application

Jerry discovered his procrastination at work actually stemmed from fear of success—worrying he'd outgrow certain relationships. Recognising that fear opened the path to discussing healthy support systems and career progress.

Worksheet 20: Identifying External vs. Internal Motivations

Title
Identifying External vs. Internal Motivations

Purpose
Clients distinguish whether they're pursuing certain goals because they truly want them (internal) or because others expect it (external). Discrepancies often arise from external pressures clashing with personal values.

The Rationale
Deci and Ryan (2008) stress the importance of self-driven (intrinsic) motivations for lasting change. Recognising extrinsic motives can clarify where resistance stems from.

Step-by-Step Instructions

1. List each major goal or pursuit.
2. Mark which ones are primarily externally driven (to please family, society) versus internally driven (personal growth, joy).
3. Explore how an externally driven approach might conflict with real preferences.
4. Consider ways to make each goal more internally meaningful or modify it if it no longer feels authentic.

Tips for Debriefing

- Affirm that external motivators aren't always negative, but intrinsic alignment fosters deeper commitment.
- Suggest partial modifications so the goal resonates more personally.

Troubleshooting Common Challenges

- If they're reluctant to label external influences, reframe it gently: "Is this mostly for you, or for someone else's expectations?"
- If they realise many goals aren't truly theirs, explore how to adapt or negotiate them.

Reflection Questions

- Which goal feels most genuinely yours?
- Could you infuse any external goal with some personal meaning?

Real life application
Keira chased a management position due to parental expectations. Recognising her real passion was creative work, she re-evaluated that path and found ways to keep growth opportunities while seeking more design tasks at her job.

Worksheet 21: Insightful Quotes

Title
Insightful Quotes

Purpose
You share brief, relevant quotes about authenticity or living according to values. The client reflects on whether these words apply to their current discrepancy, possibly gaining fresh inspiration.

The Rationale
Hill (2010) observes that concise quotes can offer aha moments. They spark reflections unachievable by simple statements of fact.

Step-by-Step Instructions

1. Provide a few short quotes (e.g., from philosophers, authors) about values, authenticity, or change.
2. Invite the client to pick one that resonates.
3. Ask how it relates to their life right now.
4. Discuss any discrepancy it highlights and how it might guide next steps.

Tips for Debriefing

- Keep quotes brief and universal.
- Encourage them to respond freely, even if they criticise a quote.

Troubleshooting Common Challenges

- If none resonates, ask them to share or find a quote they like.
- If they find quotes cliché, shift to other discrepancy tools.

Reflection Questions

- Which quote stirred something in you? Why?
- Did it hint at any change you want to pursue?

Real life application
Jamal read a line about "Courage being grace under pressure" and saw his daily avoidance as the opposite of that courage. This insight nudged him to face small fears daily rather than hide.

Worksheet 22: Empathy for the Struggle

Title
Empathy for the Struggle

Purpose
You reflect compassion for how tough it can be to keep behaviours consistent with one's ideals, reducing shame and encouraging honest acceptance.

The Rationale
Rogers (1957) highlights that unconditional positive regard can calm self-critical clients. Knowing you empathise with their struggle fosters openness to change.

Step-by-Step Instructions

1. Ask the client about the emotional toll of living in conflict with values.
2. Reflect statements like, "It must be exhausting trying to juggle these demands."
3. Reassure them they're not alone in facing these dilemmas.
4. Invite them to consider how being kind to themselves might reduce inner friction.

Tips for Debriefing

- If they express guilt, emphasise that many people experience these conflicts.
- Keep your tone steady and caring, validating their stress or embarrassment.

Troubleshooting Common Challenges

- If they respond with "I deserve this pain," gently challenge that belief or refer to another worksheet on self-compassion.
- If they shut down, accept their pace, continuing empathic reflection.

Reflection Questions

- How does it feel knowing this struggle is common?
- What could self-compassion look like in this scenario?

Real life application

Jenn felt deeply ashamed about failing to live up to her family's moral code. The therapist offered empathy, acknowledging how draining it was. Feeling understood, Jenn dared to voice deeper worries, leading to more genuine planning for improvements.

Worksheet 23: Shame vs. Guilt Discussion

Title

Shame vs. Guilt Discussion

Purpose

You clarify the difference between shame (seeing oneself as bad) and guilt (seeing a behaviour as bad). This helps the client focus on changing actions instead of condemning themselves.

The Rationale

Seligman (2011) says that shame stifles progress, while healthy guilt can motivate. Understanding this distinction reduces self-blame and fosters forward movement.

Step-by-Step Instructions

1. Define shame (global self-judgment) and guilt (specific behaviour regret).
2. Ask the client about times they felt "I am bad" versus "I did something not aligned with my values."

3. Reflect how guilt can inspire learning but shame can paralyse.
4. Encourage them to watch self-talk for each type of statement.

Tips for Debriefing

- Reassure them that seeing behaviour as changeable is more empowering than internalising shame.
- Offer strategies if shame overwhelms them (journaling, self-compassion phrases).

Troubleshooting Common Challenges

- If they're entrenched in shame, normalise those feelings while gently suggesting small steps to reframe.
- If they struggle with severe shame issues, consider deeper therapy or trauma-informed approaches.

Reflection Questions

- Which situation caused you guilt rather than shame?
- How can focusing on "this behaviour felt wrong" help you adapt?

Real life application
Michael often said, "I'm worthless." The therapist reframed it to, "You regret acting in ways that conflict with who you want to be." He began distinguishing guilt over certain choices from believing he was inherently flawed.

Worksheet 24: Creating a Personal Mission Statement

Title
Creating a Personal Mission Statement

Purpose
You support the client in drafting a concise statement of their highest ideals or life vision, then compare it to their regular choices.

The Rationale

Bandura (1997) claims that a clearly stated mission encourages consistent behaviour. Contrasting daily conduct with a personal creed often exposes areas needing adjustment.

Step-by-Step Instructions

1. Prompt them with questions: "What do you stand for?" "How do you want to be remembered?"
2. Help them shape a short mission statement (1–2 sentences).
3. Ask which current behaviours honour or contradict that statement.
4. Plan small alignment steps.

Tips for Debriefing

- Remind them it's a living statement, not set in stone.
- If they find it too grand, focus on core words or themes they resonate with.

Troubleshooting Common Challenges

- If they have trouble, brainstorm words like "respect, growth, kindness," weaving them together.
- If they consider it cheesy, encourage seeing it as a directional guide.

Reflection Questions

- How does re-reading your mission statement affect your daily decisions?
- Which part of your life do you want to align first?

Real life application

Yvonne formed the statement: "I aim to be a caring friend and lifelong learner." She noticed that constant complaining contradicted "caring," so she tried to bring more positive energy and constructive talk to her friendships.

Worksheet 25: Emotional Discrepancy Check

Title
Emotional Discrepancy Check

Purpose
You prompt clients to notice when their emotional reactions (anger, jealousy, despair) conflict with the calm or acceptance they profess to value, shedding light on internal incongruities.

The Rationale
Miller and Rollnick (2013) highlight that emotional responses can reveal hidden friction. Recognising an emotional mismatch fosters self-awareness.

Step-by-Step Instructions

1. Ask them to track strong emotions throughout the week.
2. For each, note the value or principle they believe in that the emotion challenges ("I want to be forgiving, but I felt rage").
3. Reflect on what triggered the reaction, exploring if it opposes their ideal emotional stance.
4. Encourage small practices that move them closer to the emotional style they wish to embody.

Tips for Debriefing

- Emphasise that no emotion is "bad," but it can sometimes clash with self-chosen values.
- Offer calming or grounding techniques if intense feelings surface.

Troubleshooting Common Challenges

- If they deny emotional conflict, gently invite them to consider mild cases.
- If they become upset by noticing negative feelings, reassure them it's a normal step in reconciling goals and reality.

Reflection Questions

- Which emotion do you think most clashes with the way you want to live?
- How might you handle that feeling differently next time?

Real life application

David prided himself on being patient but found himself snapping at co-workers. Realising the discrepancy, he started pausing to breathe before responding, gradually reducing outbursts that contradicted his sense of patience.

Worksheet 26: Habit-Breakdown Worksheet

Title

Habit-Breakdown Worksheet

Purpose

You pick a habit that clashes with a key value, dissecting its triggers, rewards, and cycles. This clarifies how to intervene and bring behaviour closer to personal principles.

The Rationale

Skinner (1953) and cognitive-behavioural approaches argue that understanding a habit's loop (cue, routine, reward) fosters targeted change. Clients reduce the mismatch by addressing the loop.

Step-by-Step Instructions

1. Choose a single habit.
2. Identify the trigger (time, location, emotion).
3. Note the habitual behaviour in detail.
4. Record the immediate and long-term reward or outcome.
5. Brainstorm small tweaks—altering triggers or substituting a more value-aligned routine.

Tips for Debriefing

- Remind them that even slight adjustments can disrupt an old pattern.
- Encourage focusing on one habit at a time to avoid overwhelm.

Troubleshooting Common Challenges

- If they cannot define the reward, suggest they observe carefully next time it occurs.
- If they list many triggers, pick the most common or strongest one to tackle first.

Reflection Questions

- What triggers the habit most consistently?
- How might you replace the routine with something that better fits your values?

Real life application
Francine wanted to align her eating with health values but kept snacking on sugary treats. Mapping triggers (boredom at 3 p.m.) and noticing the immediate pleasure led her to replace the snack with fruit and a quick stretching break, feeling more consistent with her health goal.

Worksheet 27: Reinforcement Analysis

Title
Reinforcement Analysis

Purpose
You investigate what the client gains or avoids by persisting in a behaviour that conflicts with their values, revealing hidden payoffs or relief that might maintain the behaviour.

The Rationale
Prochaska and DiClemente (1983) remark that even "bad" habits provide some perceived benefit, or else they'd be dropped. Identifying that benefit uncovers the real target for transformation.

Step-by-Step Instructions

1. Focus on a behaviour at odds with their ideals.
2. Ask, "What do you get out of doing it?" and "What do you avoid by doing it?"
3. Summarise the reinforcements.

4. Explore alternative ways to achieve or avoid those same things more in line with their values.

Tips for Debriefing

- Remind them that every behaviour meets a need, even if it's not healthy.
- Affirm it's a normal part of being human to seek comfort or relief.

Troubleshooting Common Challenges

- If they resist acknowledging any payoff, gently prompt about short-term ease or emotional relief.
- If they see no alternatives, brainstorm together, referencing prior successful coping.

Reflection Questions

- Which reward is hardest to give up?
- Could that need be met differently, without conflicting with your values?

Real life application
Marco's heavy video gaming clashed with his academic goals. He realised it gave instant gratification and helped him forget pressures. They discussed structured "fun breaks" and stress-management techniques that didn't hinder his studying.

Worksheet 28: Consequences for Loved Ones

Title
Consequences for Loved Ones

Purpose
You have the client reflect on how their discrepancy might affect important people in their life, increasing empathy and highlighting broader impacts.

The Rationale
Miller and Rollnick (2013) mention that seeing how loved ones are influenced can fuel

stronger motivation. People often shift once they realise they're harming or disappointing those they care about.

Step-by-Step Instructions

1. List the client's closest relationships or important figures (partner, children, friends).
2. For each, note ways that unaligned behaviour might inconvenience or hurt them.
3. Reflect how these effects measure up against the client's value of caring or loyalty.
4. Discuss possible steps to reduce negative impacts on others.

Tips for Debriefing

- Stress that this is not about shame but about empathy and connection.
- If tension arises, empathise with the guilt or grief and refocus on workable changes.

Troubleshooting Common Challenges

- If they claim it affects no one, gently ask them to consider subtle emotional or financial influences.
- If deep regret emerges, help them transform regret into constructive action.

Reflection Questions

- Which relationship do you worry about impacting the most?
- Could aligning your actions with your values improve things for them?

Real life application
Jade considered how her frequent drinking led her to cancel family visits last minute. Realising it clashed with her value of being a reliable sister, she felt encouraged to seek help controlling her alcohol use.

Worksheet 29: Empowered Reassessment

Title
Empowered Reassessment

Purpose
You invite the client to reevaluate their goals or stance now that they've learned more about their discrepancies, reinforcing that they hold the power to alter or reaffirm their aims.

The Rationale
Deci and Ryan (2008) stress autonomy and periodic reassessment to ensure the process remains self-directed, preventing forced compliance.

Step-by-Step Instructions

1. Summarise insights gained about values and mismatches so far.
2. Ask, "How do you feel about these goals now? Any changes or confirmations?"
3. Encourage them to modify or keep them if they remain true.
4. Remind them it's healthy to evolve goals as new clarity emerges.

Tips for Debriefing

- Validate that pivoting a goal or approach doesn't mean failure.
- Praise them for self-honesty, even if they decide to slow or shift direction.

Troubleshooting Common Challenges

- If they hesitate, reassure them there's no rush to finalise everything.
- If they blame external pressure for prior goals, help them craft more personally resonant ones.

Reflection Questions

- Which original goal still makes sense to you?
- Did you discover a new aim or priority?

Real life application
Larry initially aimed to quit his job for higher pay but found it clashed with a deeper love for workplace camaraderie. Reassessing, he decided to stay but request a role change, aligning better with both his need for challenge and social connection.

Worksheet 30: Finding Exceptions

Title
Finding Exceptions

Purpose
You encourage recalling moments when the client did act in harmony with their values despite past patterns, showing them their capacity for alignment.

The Rationale
Seligman (2011) contends that identifying exceptions fosters self-efficacy. If they managed alignment once, they can do it again.

Step-by-Step Instructions

1. Ask them to share an example of a day or event where they behaved entirely consistently with a core value.
2. Explore what made that scenario different.
3. Reflect which strengths or supports contributed.
4. Brainstorm how to replicate or adapt those conditions more frequently.

Tips for Debriefing

- Praise any small success they recall.
- If they find no example, let them think about partial alignments or micro-changes.

Troubleshooting Common Challenges

- If they truly see no exception, ask about any single instance of partial success.
- If they dismiss it as luck, gently highlight their role or effort.

Reflection Questions

- What did that successful moment teach you about yourself?
- How could you recreate some of those conditions in daily life?

Real life application
Paula thought she'd never gone a week without overspending but remembered once saving for a holiday. Realising she can manage finances under motivational deadlines, she set smaller short-term saving goals to keep momentum.

Worksheet 31: Uncovering Hidden Values

Title
Uncovering Hidden Values

Purpose
You use open-ended exploration to identify values the client might not realise they hold, widening the lens on how their behaviour might be out of step with deeper beliefs.

The Rationale
Miller and Rollnick (2013) suggest that some clients haven't fully named or owned certain values, so surfacing them can heighten discrepancy awareness.

Step-by-Step Instructions

1. Ask broad prompts: "What qualities do you admire in others?" "What do you stand against?"
2. Note any repeated themes (fairness, kindness, truth).
3. Reflect these potential hidden values back to them.
4. See if their daily routines or decisions line up or clash with these newly realised values.

Tips for Debriefing

- Remind them it's okay to discover values they never spoke of before.
- Offer gentle validation if they feel surprised or emotional about these insights.

Troubleshooting Common Challenges

- If they claim no strong beliefs, mention smaller ideals like courtesy or reliability.
- If they show confusion, let them sit with partial thoughts to refine later.

Reflection Questions

- Which newly acknowledged value resonates with you most strongly?
- How do you see it shaping your future choices?

Real life application

Shaun admired people who always kept their word. Realising he valued loyalty, he saw how frequently he'd bail on commitments last-minute. This insight propelled him to plan better to uphold loyalty in his schedule.

Worksheet 32: Appreciating Progress

Title

Appreciating Progress

Purpose

You highlight any small steps or partial improvements toward living in line with values, reinforcing positivity and sustaining momentum.

The Rationale

Rogers (1957) underscores that celebrating incremental progress cements motivation and reduces the sense of inadequacy.

Step-by-Step Instructions

1. Ask them to recall any minor effort, even just noticing a discrepancy or resisting an old pattern once.
2. Reflect how this attempt or awareness is a sign of growth.
3. Discuss how it felt to take that small step.
4. Explore how to build on these successes.

Tips for Debriefing

- Ensure the praise is specific: point out exactly what they did well.
- If they brush it off as trivial, gently emphasise that big changes start with small seeds.

Troubleshooting Common Challenges

- If they can't see progress, mention anything you've observed in sessions (like a more open attitude).
- If they're perfectionistic, remind them that partial success is still success.

Reflection Questions

- Which small win do you feel proud of this week?
- How might you expand that change into another aspect of your daily life?

Real life application
Brittany found she spoke up once in a meeting where she used to stay silent, aligning with her value of assertiveness. She initially dismissed it as minor, but realising it was a meaningful shift encouraged her to keep speaking up.

Worksheet 33: Visual Cues

Title
Visual Cues

Purpose
You suggest physical reminders (quotes, symbols) in the client's environment to prompt recall of their top values and highlight the gap whenever they slip into old patterns.

The Rationale
Bandura (1997) indicates that frequent prompts maintain a sense of accountability to personal aims. When a visual cue appears, it nudges reflection and self-correction.

Step-by-Step Instructions

1. Collaborate on a short list of visual tokens (a note on the mirror, a motivational wallpaper, a bracelet).
2. Ensure each item references a specific value or a small positive statement.
3. Encourage them to place or wear it in a location they'll frequently see.
4. Ask them to observe any shift in behaviour or mindset triggered by the reminders.

Tips for Debriefing

- If they prefer minimal fuss, start with just one cue in a key spot.
- Remind them to update or rotate cues if they become too familiar and lose impact.

Troubleshooting Common Challenges

- If they find it embarrassing at first, suggest discreet cues (phone background, coded bracelet).
- If they ignore the cues, prompt them to reflect on why.

Reflection Questions

- Which type of visual reminder resonates with you the most?
- How do you react when you see it in a challenging moment?

Real life application
Derek placed a small sticky note reading "Health Over Haste" on his fridge. Each time he was tempted to grab junk food quickly, he paused to recall his value of better nutrition, gradually choosing healthier snacks.

Worksheet 34: Compare and Contrast

Title
Compare and Contrast

Purpose
You invite the client to envision two paths: continuing current behaviour versus

344

aligning with values. Juxtaposing these scenarios can clarify potential trade-offs and gains.

The Rationale

Prochaska and DiClemente (1983) suggest side-by-side comparisons help clients weigh real pros and cons, often motivating them to pick the path that better suits their aspirations.

Step-by-Step Instructions

1. Draw two columns: "If I keep on this track…" and "If I shift to value-aligned choices…"
2. Fill in likely daily experiences, emotional states, or relationship outcomes for each.
3. Compare them. Notice which path sounds more fulfilling or consistent with deeper ideals.
4. Reflect on small steps to move from one column to the other.

Tips for Debriefing

- Encourage honesty; the first column might have some short-term comforts.
- Remind them no solution is perfect, but alignment often yields longer-term satisfaction.

Troubleshooting Common Challenges

- If they see only negatives in changing, reflect on possible overlooked positives.
- If they see both columns as equally unappealing, focus on partial modifications or a different goal.

Reflection Questions

- Which column ultimately feels more aligned with your best future?
- Can you see a middle path if extremes feel too distant?

Real life application

Carla wrote that continuing to ignore her finances might yield short-term fun but lead to deeper debt stress. Aligning with her value of responsibility meant some sacrifices now but a calmer future. Comparing them reinforced her resolve to budget.

Worksheet 35: Identifying Conflicting Needs

Title
Identifying Conflicting Needs

Purpose
You help clients see if their discrepancy springs from competing needs (e.g., the need for security vs. the need for freedom). Recognising these drives can help them find a balanced approach.

The Rationale
Egan (2013) notes that conflict often arises when multiple core needs compete. Understanding them clarifies how to satisfy both in ways that reduce the gap.

Step-by-Step Instructions

1. Ask, "Which personal needs might be pushing you in opposite directions?"
2. List each need (e.g., social connection vs. privacy, stability vs. novelty).
3. Reflect how these opposing needs create tension.
4. Brainstorm strategies to honour each in moderate ways.

Tips for Debriefing

- Validate that having multiple needs is natural and can lead to ambivalence.
- Suggest testing small compromises to see if both needs get some satisfaction.

Troubleshooting Common Challenges

- If they claim they must pick one need over all others, explore partial fulfilment or flexible scheduling.
- If they blame external demands, reflect on how internal desires also factor in.

Reflection Questions

- Which pair of conflicting needs challenges you most?
- Could a middle path reduce stress while meeting both needs enough?

Real life application
Mark craved freedom but also felt a deep need for family closeness. He chose to plan one weekend a month for solo adventures while dedicating the rest to consistent family time, balancing both.

Worksheet 36: Refining Long-Term Goals

Title
Refining Long-Term Goals

Purpose
Clients might find their long-term aims too big or too vague. You refine them into clearer, more tangible targets, revealing any mismatch with daily choices.

The Rationale
Bandura (1997) shows that precise goals aid self-efficacy. Vague dreams can perpetuate confusion and conflict.

Step-by-Step Instructions

1. Have the client list major future goals.
2. Ensure each is concrete: "Save £5,000 in a year," "Run a 5K," not just "be secure" or "get fit."
3. Check if daily routines align with these refined goals.
4. Note any contradictions that need to be addressed.

Tips for Debriefing

- Remind them to be specific and use approximate timelines or measurable markers.
- If a goal is huge, break it down (linked to Worksheet 3 on cost-benefit or Worksheet 11's analysis).

Troubleshooting Common Challenges

- If they insist on broad goals, gently highlight how specifics bolster clarity.

- If they worry about failing a big target, offer stepping stones or shorter intervals.

Reflection Questions

- Which refined goal energises you?
- Are your daily habits geared to meet it?

Real life application

Dana changed "I want better finances" to "I want to pay off £2,000 of credit card debt in 6 months." She noticed her weekly spending contradicted that. Aiming for specifics made her track and curb unnecessary expenses.

Worksheet 37: Discrepancy Dialogue

Title

Discrepancy Dialogue

Purpose

You propose a short role-play where the client acts out an internal dialogue between the part that wants to uphold values and the part that resists, exposing the tension clearly.

The Rationale

Miller and Rollnick (2013) highlight that letting both sides speak can be enlightening, showing the internal push-pull that maintains the gap.

Step-by-Step Instructions

1. Ask the client to choose two "voices": Value-Driven Self vs. Resistant Self.
2. Let them voice each perspective in turn, capturing the main arguments.
3. Reflect or paraphrase after each "side" speaks.
4. End by discussing any new understanding or compromise.

Tips for Debriefing

- Encourage them to adopt different tones or postures for each voice if comfortable.
- Remind them this is a safe exercise—no right answer is forced.

Troubleshooting Common Challenges

- If they feel silly, keep it brief or do it in writing.
- If conflict escalates, remind them the goal is insight, not winning an internal argument.

Reflection Questions

- Did letting each side speak help you see their needs?
- Which voice do you feel drawn to after hearing both?

Real life application
Sue's "health-focused voice" pleaded for consistent workouts, while her "lazy voice" insisted on comfort. Hearing them out made Sue notice she needed gentler exercise routines to ease into a habit, addressing both comfort and health.

Worksheet 38: Self-Compassion Reminders

Title
Self-Compassion Reminders

Purpose
In times when they realise they're not following their values, you encourage them to practise a brief self-compassion approach, preventing shame and focusing on constructive improvement.

The Rationale
Neff (2011) underlines the power of self-compassion in bridging discrepancies. Rather than self-attack, kind self-talk fosters positive change.

Step-by-Step Instructions

1. Brainstorm short phrases they can say (e.g., "I messed up, but I can learn and do better," or "I'm allowed to make mistakes while striving to improve").
2. Ask them to practise these lines whenever they spot a mismatch.
3. Reflect on how each phrase influences their emotional state.
4. Keep track of changes in how they respond to slip-ups.

Tips for Debriefing

- If they find self-kindness hard, remind them they'd likely offer compassion to a friend in the same position.
- Encourage them to keep a note in their phone or wallet as a prompt.

Troubleshooting Common Challenges

- If they dismiss this as weak or silly, reframe it: it takes courage to show kindness to oneself.
- If negative self-talk is severe, combine this with more in-depth therapy strategies.

Reflection Questions

- Which self-compassion phrase feels most comforting or believable?
- How might that acceptance help you stay motivated?

Real life application
Olivia repeated, "I can learn from this slip-up," after she broke her vow to limit online shopping. Instead of spiralling into guilt, she calmly revised her budget plan, noticing the difference in mood and resilience.

Worksheet 39: Monitoring Alignment Daily

Title
Monitoring Alignment Daily

Purpose
Clients rate each day on how closely they lived by their values, writing a short reason.

This ongoing awareness fosters conscious choices and reveals improvement or stagnation.

The Rationale

Seligman (2011) shows that frequent self-monitoring consolidates mindful behaviour. A daily reflection keeps them in tune with their integrity goals.

Step-by-Step Instructions

1. Give them a simple daily chart: columns for "Date," "Alignment Score (1–10)," "Why?"
2. Each evening, they pick a number showing how well they adhered to core principles.
3. They note a brief explanation: "I avoided gossip today" or "I argued with my spouse out of anger."
4. Review weekly or monthly, celebrating increments of progress.

Tips for Debriefing

- Remind them not to judge themselves harshly; it's a reflection tool.
- Keep it quick so it's not a chore: a 30-second check each night is enough.

Troubleshooting Common Challenges

- If they forget, suggest a phone reminder or keep the chart visible.
- If they see no improvement, gently discuss patterns or triggers; reaffirm patience.

Reflection Questions

- Did you notice any pattern about days with higher alignment scores?
- How did writing a daily reason help clarify your ups and downs?

Real life application

Jon used a nightly alignment log. When he rated 9/10 one day, he credited it to finishing tasks on time and showing kindness to colleagues. This positive feedback loop motivated repeating those actions.

Worksheet 40: Reflecting Movement Toward Harmony

Title
Reflecting Movement Toward Harmony

Purpose
You periodically summarise any shifts toward the client's chosen ideals, reinforcing those changes and emphasising that bridging the gap is possible.

The Rationale
Miller and Rollnick (2013) show that acknowledging even slight forward steps cements belief in eventual success, encouraging continued effort.

Step-by-Step Instructions

1. Occasionally ask them to recall improvements they've made or insights gained regarding living by their values.
2. Reflect these achievements clearly: "You once avoided setting boundaries, now you speak up politely."
3. Validate how it feels to reduce the gap, even if just a little.
4. Ask if they want to refine or expand the next step.

Tips for Debriefing

- Tie progress back to initial motivations or goals.
- Suggest repeating the process: noticing small gains can accumulate over time.

Troubleshooting Common Challenges

- If they claim minimal progress, remind them of small changes in attitude or new problem-solving skills.
- If they backslide, emphasise that one slip doesn't invalidate prior strides.

Reflection Questions

- Which change so far gives you the most satisfaction?
- How could you push just a bit further on that front?

Real life application
After months of gradual changes, Annie looked back: she'd cut her nightly wine from three glasses to one and joined a painting class to honour her creative side. Hearing the therapist reflect these improvements motivated her to keep going.

Goal Setting and Planning

This set directs the client to structure specific, achievable aims. Worksheets cover breaking down bigger objectives into manageable tasks, scheduling actions, and reviewing feasibility. Clearly defined steps, timelines, and success markers keep the individual organised and inspired.

Worksheet 1: Brainstorm Potential Paths

Title
Brainstorm Potential Paths

Purpose
You help the client tap into creativity and list multiple possibilities for reaching their goal. This open exploration expands options before tightening the plan.

The Rationale
Miller and Rollnick (2013) indicate that brainstorming can free clients from rigid thinking and reveal surprising routes to success. Exploring many paths reduces the chance of feeling cornered by a single approach.

Step-by-Step Instructions

1. Invite the client to write down or say any idea—big or small—for achieving the main target.
2. Encourage wild or unconventional thoughts without judging feasibility yet.
3. Reflect each idea, noticing the energy behind it.
4. Save all ideas for further narrowing in upcoming steps.

Tips for Debriefing

- Let them know there are no bad suggestions in brainstorming; quantity is the aim.
- Show enthusiasm for each idea to foster a sense of creativity.

Troubleshooting Common Challenges

- If they hesitate, ask them to imagine how friends or role models might solve the problem.
- If they get stuck, consider breaking it into categories like "short-term," "bold leaps," and "in-between."

Reflection Questions

- Which idea, even if it seems wild, are you drawn to?

- How did it feel to set aside judgment and imagine freely?

Real life application
Sean brainstormed ways to handle stress at work. He listed everything from changing departments to taking a mid-day walk. Although some ideas seemed unlikely, it revealed fresh options that lit a spark of excitement.

Worksheet 2: SMART Goal Drafting

Title
SMART Goal Drafting

Purpose
You convert the client's vision into one or two clear SMART goals—Specific, Measurable, Achievable, Relevant, Time-bound—so the outcome feels concrete and trackable.

The Rationale
Bandura (1997) found that specific, well-defined goals enhance self-belief. By sharpening a broad desire into SMART form, motivation grows and success becomes more likely.

Step-by-Step Instructions

1. Pick one promising idea from the brainstorming stage.
2. Break it down into SMART language: exact result, how to measure, realism check, personal relevance, and a deadline.
3. Write the final statement.
4. Review it aloud to ensure it sounds motivating yet feasible.

Tips for Debriefing

- Stress that each component matters: a vague aim or no deadline can undermine follow-through.
- Encourage them to refine the wording until it feels truly theirs.

Troubleshooting Common Challenges

- If they find it too rigid, remind them they can adjust it as they learn more.
- If they set an unrealistic time frame, guide them to break it into smaller increments.

Reflection Questions

- What part of the SMART format did you find toughest?
- Do you feel excited or daunted by this new clarity?

Real life application
Maria's goal "save money" became "Save £200 monthly for 5 months to fund a short training course, starting this week." This specificity helped her track each deposit confidently.

Worksheet 3: Action Step Breakdown

Title
Action Step Breakdown

Purpose
You reduce a broad goal into a list of tiny tasks, showing clear progression from start to finish. This minimises overwhelm and clarifies the path forward.

The Rationale
Miller and Rollnick (2013) argue that subdividing goals helps clients see each stage as doable. Momentum builds as they tick off smaller tasks.

Step-by-Step Instructions

1. Begin with your newly formed SMART goal.
2. Brainstorm every required action (gather materials, schedule practice, etc.).
3. Order them logically: easiest or earliest steps first, more demanding tasks next.
4. Note estimated time or resources for each step.

Tips for Debriefing

- Applaud the client for noticing small but essential details.
- Remind them to keep the list flexible—some tasks might overlap or reorder as they progress.

Troubleshooting Common Challenges

- If the list gets too long, group tasks into categories.
- If they skip vital steps, gently prompt them to think of any dependencies.

Reflection Questions

- Which step feels most urgent to do first?
- Which step do you anticipate being the hardest?

Real life application

Adil aimed to launch a small web store. He listed steps: research products, open a merchant account, design a logo, create item listings, and plan shipping methods. Seeing it all laid out eased his anxiety about missing key tasks.

Worksheet 4: Plan Feasibility Check

Title

Plan Feasibility Check

Purpose

You examine whether each proposed action step suits the client's real-life constraints (time, money, energy). Adjusting early saves frustration later.

The Rationale

Prochaska and DiClemente (1983) underscore that realistic plans foster adherence. Screening for feasibility at the outset prevents a meltdown mid-process.

Step-by-Step Instructions

1. Review the action steps from the breakdown.
2. For each, ask the client to estimate difficulty level and required resources.
3. Adjust time frames or scale tasks down if anything seems unmanageable.
4. Finalise an updated plan that fits the client's capacity and schedule.

Tips for Debriefing

- Validate their limits: no one can do it all instantly.
- Check for emotional energy as well as physical or financial resources.

Troubleshooting Common Challenges

- If they repeatedly claim "I can handle it," gently confirm they have enough support or buffer time.
- If they feel discouraged by cutbacks, reframe it as strategic pacing.

Reflection Questions

- Which step currently feels the biggest stretch?
- How can you balance ambition with reality?

Real life application
Tessa wanted to practice guitar every night, but after the feasibility check, she limited it to four nights since her job included late shifts. This adjustment prevented burnout and helped her stick to the plan consistently.

Worksheet 5: Calendar Scheduling

Title
Calendar Scheduling

Purpose
You have the client place their action steps into a real schedule, ensuring tasks don't remain abstract. This fosters time management and accountability.

The Rationale

Skinner (1953) indicates that linking behaviour to specific cues—like day and time—reduces forgetting or procrastination. A written schedule clarifies commitment.

Step-by-Step Instructions

1. Pick a calendar format the client prefers (digital, paper).
2. Insert each step from the feasible plan with dates and times.
3. Encourage adding reminders or alarms.
4. Double-check that tasks are spaced realistically.

Tips for Debriefing

- If they're new to scheduling, show them how to block specific intervals.
- Suggest building in buffer zones in case tasks run longer.

Troubleshooting Common Challenges

- If they're resistant to a rigid timetable, compromise with weekly goals in a flexible window.
- If their schedule is chaotic, help them prioritise top tasks first.

Reflection Questions

- Which day or time slot do you see as a natural fit for these tasks?
- How will you handle unexpected disruptions?

Real life application

Glenn used his phone's calendar to slot 30-minute sessions for job application tasks on Mondays and Wednesdays. Setting alerts increased follow-through, turning vague intentions into consistent effort.

Worksheet 6: Risk Assessment

Title

Risk Assessment

Purpose
You look at potential pitfalls or obstacles for each step, preparing solutions in advance. This lowers the chance of being derailed by unforeseen problems.

The Rationale
Miller and Rollnick (2013) propose identifying vulnerabilities early fosters resilience. Predicting issues helps manage them calmly rather than reacting in crisis mode.

Step-by-Step Instructions

1. For every major step in the plan, list likely challenges (lack of time, cost, emotional distress).
2. Brainstorm ways to counter or minimise each risk.
3. Document a short backup approach: "If X happens, I'll do Y."
4. If any risk feels severe, explore how to reduce it further or find external help.

Tips for Debriefing

- Normalise that all goals face setbacks. Planning is a sign of strength, not pessimism.
- Stress that having a fallback can boost confidence.

Troubleshooting Common Challenges

- If the client sees no risks, gently prompt them about known stressors or past obstacles.
- If they become anxious listing problems, remind them this is proactive, not negativity.

Reflection Questions

- Which risk concerns you most?
- What do you see as a practical first response if that risk appears?

Real life application
Aria knew that heavy workloads might prevent her from daily exercise. She decided if her schedule was overrun, she'd do 10-minute HIIT workouts at home instead of hitting the gym for an hour, maintaining momentum.

Worksheet 7: Progress Metric Design

Title
Progress Metric Design

Purpose
You define how the client will measure progress—through checklists, rating scales, logs, or apps—keeping them motivated and aware of each step forward.

The Rationale
Bandura (1997) suggests that visible evidence of improvement reinforces self-belief. Good metrics help track real gains rather than subjective impressions alone.

Step-by-Step Instructions

1. Discuss with the client which format suits them: daily checklists, weekly self-ratings, or a digital tracker.
2. Decide on frequency (daily, thrice a week, etc.).
3. Keep it simple—only measure the key items that indicate genuine movement.
4. Preview how they'll review and revise these metrics as needed.

Tips for Debriefing

- Encourage them not to measure everything if that feels overwhelming. Focus on crucial indicators.
- Affirm they can switch tools if one doesn't motivate them.

Troubleshooting Common Challenges

- If they resist data tracking, ask them how they'll notice small wins.
- If they over-measure and stress out, narrow it to the most important items.

Reflection Questions

- Which progress indicator will feel most rewarding to watch?
- How might tracking results change your daily choices?

Real life application

Mike designed a daily water intake log on his phone plus a weekly weigh-in to watch health improvements. Seeing small increments in water consumption gave him confidence he was on the right track.

Worksheet 8: Accountability Structure

Title

Accountability Structure

Purpose

You decide how the client wishes to remain accountable—through scheduled updates, peer support, or self-monitoring—ensuring they stay on track.

The Rationale

Prochaska and DiClemente (1983) emphasise that a supportive system can prevent relapse. Consistent check-ins can keep clients focused despite busy routines or doubts.

Step-by-Step Instructions

1. Ask them to choose an accountability format (a weekly text to a friend, monthly call with a mentor, or using an online group).
2. Define frequency and type of update: progress reports, shared achievements, or logs.
3. Clarify if they prefer a formal or casual approach.
4. Mark the chosen accountability plan in the calendar or progress tracker.

Tips for Debriefing

- Let them tailor it to their comfort—some prefer discreet check-ins, others need group dynamics.
- Applaud them for seeking outside support, a sign of determination, not weakness.

Troubleshooting Common Challenges

- If they're shy about involving others, suggest gentle digital check-ins or an anonymous forum.
- If they fear judgement from peers, pick a supportive friend or professional who fosters positivity.

Reflection Questions

- Who could you rely on to cheer you on or keep you honest?
- How do you feel about giving someone regular updates?

Real life application
Fiona decided to send a brief Sunday night text to her sister, reporting whether she met her writing goal that week. Anticipating the check-in motivated her to prioritise writing slots, as she hated to admit zero progress.

Worksheet 9: Reward System

Title
Reward System

Purpose
You help the client outline small, meaningful rewards for hitting milestones, reinforcing each success and adding fun to the journey.

The Rationale
Skinner (1953) states that positive reinforcement cements habits. Tangible or experiential treats can keep motivation high when goals get tough.

Step-by-Step Instructions

1. Ask them to list low-cost, enjoyable treats (favourite snack, extra leisure, a small gift).
2. Attach each reward to a specific milestone (e.g., finishing the first five tasks).
3. Keep the reward scale proportional—bigger achievements can merit bigger treats.
4. Encourage them to actually follow through on these celebrations.

Tips for Debriefing

- Stress that rewards needn't be expensive or complicated.
- Mention intangible rewards like a relaxing bath or a social outing with a friend.

Troubleshooting Common Challenges

- If they feel guilty "indulging," reframe it as earned recognition for hard work.
- If they fear overindulgence, set boundaries (like one small treat, not an entire spree).

Reflection Questions

- Which reward excites you most and makes you want to reach that milestone?
- Do you prefer immediate small rewards or bigger ones after major targets?

Real life application

Denise decided that each time she completed her bi-weekly workout streak, she'd treat herself to a new eBook. Celebrating small wins helped sustain her motivation even on low-energy days.

Worksheet 10: Confidence Builder Steps

Title
Confidence Builder Steps

Purpose
You structure the plan so the client starts with easier tasks, gradually tackling harder ones. This builds self-assurance and momentum early on.

The Rationale
Bandura (1997) suggests that early success at simpler tasks raises self-efficacy, fueling bravery for bigger goals. Avoiding immediate large challenges prevents early discouragement.

Step-by-Step Instructions

1. Rank the tasks by difficulty.
2. Begin with the easiest or least intimidating action.
3. Slowly progress to moderate and then challenging tasks.
4. Reflect on each success to reinforce optimism.

Tips for Debriefing

- Celebrate every small achievement as a stepping stone.
- If the client's confidence is already high, ensure you're not oversimplifying. A moderate start can keep them engaged.

Troubleshooting Common Challenges

- If they want to jump straight to the biggest step, caution them about potential setbacks.
- If they get bored with easy tasks, accelerate to a mid-level challenge.

Reflection Questions

- Which first step do you feel comfortable starting tomorrow?
- How might small victories encourage you to face tougher tasks soon?

Real life application
Rohan wanted to speak publicly but was terrified. His first step was practicing alone for a few minutes each day. Feeling success there led him to present to close friends, eventually building courage for a real audience.

Worksheet 11: Incorporating Self-Care

Title
Incorporating Self-Care

Purpose
You weave self-care activities into the action plan, preventing burnout and ensuring the client maintains balance as they chase goals.

The Rationale

Miller and Rollnick (2013) emphasise that sustained effort requires replenishment. Without rest and enjoyment, motivation can collapse under stress.

Step-by-Step Instructions

1. Have them list self-care ideas (stretching breaks, hobby time, journalling).
2. Insert these items into the schedule at intervals.
3. Remind them self-care is not optional but a key part of consistent progress.
4. Revisit how each self-care activity affects energy and mood.

Tips for Debriefing

- Highlight that personal well-being supports overall success.
- If they feel guilty about "me-time," compare how a well-rested mind is better for productivity.

Troubleshooting Common Challenges

- If they say "no time," look for small slots (5-minute relaxation).
- If they find it frivolous, show them how stress reduction can boost focus.

Reflection Questions

- Which self-care practice recharges you the most?
- How will you ensure you don't skip it when busy?

Real life application

Daniel inserted a 10-minute break daily for calm breathing and music. He noticed he faced the next tasks with clearer concentration, realising self-care actually advanced his goals by keeping him sharp.

Worksheet 12: Support Network Worksheet

Title

Support Network Worksheet

Purpose
You map out who can offer emotional or practical help. This fosters a sense of community backing, making challenges more manageable.

The Rationale
Rogers (1957) found that unconditional positive regard often extends beyond therapy. Having supportive friends, family, or mentors can strengthen perseverance.

Step-by-Step Instructions

1. List people who might support, from close friends to online communities.
2. Clarify what each person can provide—emotional cheerleading, resources, skill-sharing.
3. Reach out or form a plan for how and when to involve each support.
4. Note any gaps in the network and brainstorm ways to fill them.

Tips for Debriefing

- Encourage gratitude toward these allies.
- If the client is isolated, suggest community groups or safe online forums to expand their circle.

Troubleshooting Common Challenges

- If they feel a fear of burdening others, highlight how people are often glad to help.
- If trust is an issue, start with the most reliable or professional supports.

Reflection Questions

- Who in your life has shown genuine interest in your progress?
- How might you ask for help in a way that feels comfortable?

Real life application
Tammy identified her cousin for pep talks, a local coworker for accountability, and an online forum for book recommendations. Each offered different types of motivation, preventing Tammy from feeling alone.

Worksheet 13: Environment Audit

Title
Environment Audit

Purpose
You assess how the client's surroundings (home, workspace, digital habits) help or hinder progress. Adjusting these spaces can smooth the path to success.

The Rationale
Skinner (1953) notes that environmental cues strongly shape behaviour. Tweaking routines or physical setups can reduce friction and temptation.

Step-by-Step Instructions

1. Ask them to scan their daily environments—bedroom, kitchen, phone apps—for triggers or distractions.
2. List elements that support the goal (alarm reminders, a tidy desk) vs. those that derail (junk food in plain sight, constant social media).
3. Plan minor changes (rearrange items, limit phone notifications) to encourage goal-related actions.

Tips for Debriefing

- Keep solutions simple: a post-it note, a rearranged shelf can have a big effect.
- Affirm that environment changes complement but don't replace self-discipline.

Troubleshooting Common Challenges

- If they share a living space and can't fully rearrange, brainstorm partial solutions.
- If they can't remove all temptations, focus on reducing easy access.

Reflection Questions

- Which environmental tweak would have the largest positive effect?
- How might you keep your environment supportive in the long run?

Real life application

Luke discovered leaving his phone on silent and out of reach while writing boosted concentration. He also placed his guitar in the living area, reminding him to practise. The environment now nudged him toward creative work.

Worksheet 14: Mindset Preparation

Title

Mindset Preparation

Purpose

You encourage the client to adopt affirmations or mental routines that cultivate optimism and resilience before confronting challenging tasks.

The Rationale

Seligman (2011) highlights the role of positive expectancy in tackling difficulties. An encouraging mindset paves the way for steady action.

Step-by-Step Instructions

1. Invite them to craft short, personalised statements they can repeat or read before starting a task (e.g., "I can handle new challenges").
2. Suggest quick mental or breathing exercises if they're anxious.
3. Set a routine: before each step, pause, recite or reflect on these affirmations.
4. Track how it influences performance or mood.

Tips for Debriefing

- Emphasise authenticity: pick words that truly resonate with their style, not generic phrases.
- If they doubt positivity, reframe it as a balanced approach—acknowledging obstacles but believing in effort.

Troubleshooting Common Challenges

- If they laugh off affirmations, propose subtle reminders or humour-laced statements.
- If negative self-talk persists, reinforce focusing on one uplifting phrase at a time.

Reflection Questions

- Which affirmation or pep talk line feels most genuine?
- Did any mental shift help you start tasks more calmly?

Real life application
Rita decided her phrase was, "I'm making progress, one step at a time," repeated each morning before tackling her daily steps. She reported feeling more confident as the day began.

Worksheet 15: Time-Blocking Experiment

Title
Time-Blocking Experiment

Purpose
You suggest the client assign dedicated blocks for goal-related tasks, testing a structured approach to scheduling that can heighten focus.

The Rationale
Prochaska and DiClemente (1983) found that scheduling tasks into specific time slots increases completion rates. It's a practical antidote to vague "I'll do it later" thinking.

Step-by-Step Instructions

1. Identify a set number of hours or half-hours each week for the goal activity.
2. Block them on the calendar (digital or paper).
3. Encourage them to treat these blocks as appointments not to be casually cancelled.
4. After a week, review what worked or didn't, adjusting as necessary.

Tips for Debriefing

- Mention this approach may feel unusual at first; regular check-ins can refine it.
- If they skip a block, reflect kindly on the cause and plan better for next time.

Troubleshooting Common Challenges

- If their schedule is unpredictable, consider daily or weekly planning, adjusting blocks 24 hours in advance.
- If they fear rigidity, remind them blocks can shift as long as they remain consistent.

Reflection Questions

- Did time-blocking help you avoid distractions?
- Which block felt most productive or peaceful?

Real life application
Naomi devoted 7-8 p.m. on weekdays to study for her certification exam. Treating it like a real appointment reduced the likelihood of her pushing it aside for TV or phone calls.

Worksheet 16: Commitment Contract

Title
Commitment Contract

Purpose
You guide clients to draft a brief written pact—official or informal—stating their goal, timeline, and core reasons for pursuing it. This document can enhance dedication and serve as a tangible reminder.

The Rationale
Miller and Rollnick (2013) show that personal commitment statements can reinforce motivation, especially if displayed somewhere visible or shared with a trusted ally.

Step-by-Step Instructions

1. Help them phrase a contract: "I (name) commit to (goal), by (timeframe), because (motivating reasons)."
2. Suggest they sign and date it.
3. Optionally, share it with an accountability partner or keep it somewhere seen daily.
4. Revisit or update the contract if the goal evolves.

Tips for Debriefing

- Stress that it's a personal contract, not a source of guilt if difficulties arise.
- If they worry about pressure, let them include a clause about flexibility.

Troubleshooting Common Challenges

- If they don't like the formal feel, they can phrase it more casually or artistically.
- If they fear shame, emphasise it as an encouraging symbol, not a harsh rulebook.

Reflection Questions

- What key reasons did you include for doing this?
- Where will you place your contract so it remains impactful?

Real life application
Vivian wrote a short contract: "I, Vivian, commit to finishing my novel's first draft by 1 December, driven by my passion for storytelling." Placing it on her desk kept her momentum high.

Worksheet 17: Visualization of Success

Title
Visualization of Success

Purpose
You encourage a regular mental picture where the client sees themselves achieving the goal, reinforcing positivity and problem-solving mindsets.

The Rationale
Bandura (1997) notes that mental rehearsal fosters a sense of familiarity with success, reducing fear of the unknown. This technique can strengthen perseverance.

Step-by-Step Instructions

1. Ask them to close their eyes or quietly reflect on a scene where they've completed the goal.
2. Include sensory details—sights, sounds, how they celebrate.
3. Suggest daily or weekly repetition of this short visualisation.
4. Discuss any insights or fresh motivation that emerges.

Tips for Debriefing

- Emphasise authenticity; they can tweak the scenario to feel truly meaningful.
- Keep it brief so it's easy to do frequently.

Troubleshooting Common Challenges

- If they dismiss it as daydreaming, remind them it's a psychological tool for motivation.
- If negative images intrude, normalise it and gently refocus on possible solutions.

Reflection Questions

- How do you feel when picturing your successful future self?
- Which part of the mental scene is most vivid?

Real life application
Jon pictured himself feeling confident after completing a triathlon. He visualised crossing the finish line, hearing cheers from friends. That mental scene boosted his drive to stick with training sessions.

Worksheet 18: Micro-Habits

Title
Micro-Habits

Purpose
You encourage clients to integrate tiny daily steps that, over time, accumulate into major behavioural shifts. This reduces intimidation and fosters consistency.

The Rationale
Skinner (1953) suggests that tiny, easily repeatable actions lower resistance. Achieving them daily builds momentum and forms longer-lasting routines.

Step-by-Step Instructions

1. Identify a bigger habit they want to cultivate.
2. Shrink it to a "micro" version—just one minute or simple reps.
3. Embed it in an existing routine (right after brushing teeth, for instance).
4. Track how it evolves or if it naturally expands after a few weeks.

Tips for Debriefing

- Praise even minimal success because the aim is to anchor the behaviour.
- Encourage them to gradually increase time or intensity when it feels natural.

Troubleshooting Common Challenges

- If they skip a micro-habit, check if it's still too hard or the timing is inconvenient.
- If they become overly ambitious, remind them the key is consistency, not immediate intensity.

Reflection Questions

- Which small daily action can you see yourself doing without fail?
- How might that single step grow into a bigger pattern?

Real life application

Alex wanted to start reading more, but never found time. He committed to just two pages each night after dinner. Soon two pages grew to ten, and he finished two books in a month.

Worksheet 19: Identifying High-Impact Actions

Title
Identifying High-Impact Actions

Purpose
You help the client locate tasks that produce the biggest results or breakthroughs, guiding them to prioritise these for maximum efficiency.

The Rationale
Miller and Rollnick (2013) emphasise that focusing on essential actions can yield swifter gains. Some steps matter more than others to accelerate progress.

Step-by-Step Instructions

1. From the action breakdown, star the tasks that you both believe will strongly advance the goal.
2. Order them by potential impact.
3. Plan to tackle or reinforce these "high-impact" tasks first.
4. Revisit the list occasionally to ensure they stay front and centre.

Tips for Debriefing

- Remind them they can't do everything at once, so focusing on vital steps is wise.
- Balance these tasks with smaller activities that maintain momentum.

Troubleshooting Common Challenges

- If they choose only big tasks, check feasibility so they don't burn out.

- If they avoid these tasks out of fear, explore ways to scale them down or add supportive structures.

Reflection Questions

- Which action feels most powerful for your goal?
- How will focusing on it help other tasks fall into place?

Real life application
Nadia saw that her biggest step for launching a blog was posting a first article—opening the door to future posts. Once she prioritised finishing that article, confidence grew to handle other tasks like design and promotion.

Worksheet 20: Backup Plans

Title
Backup Plans

Purpose
You develop alternative routes for each main step, maintaining progress if the original plan hits a roadblock. This fosters resilience and reduces panic.

The Rationale
Prochaska and DiClemente (1983) remind us that obstacles are normal. Having a Plan B (or C) can preserve morale, ensuring momentum doesn't collapse at the first setback.

Step-by-Step Instructions

1. List each crucial step from the plan.
2. Brainstorm a fallback method for each, e.g., if gym visits fail, switch to home workouts.
3. Write these backups next to the primary step.
4. Stress that switching to a backup is a smart adaptation, not a failure.

Tips for Debriefing

- Normalise that real life is unpredictable; pivoting is a sign of strength.
- Encourage them to keep an open mind if the backup starts working better than the original idea.

Troubleshooting Common Challenges

- If they fear too many "what ifs," reassure them that a single backup is enough—no need to over-plan.
- If they never use the primary plan because backups feel easier, gently revisit their reasons for the main route.

Reflection Questions

- Which potential obstacle worries you most?
- How might you keep a balanced view of switching to a backup?

Real life application
Pierre planned daily Spanish practice using an app. If his phone malfunctioned or he lost internet, his backup was using a short textbook and audio recordings. Knowing he had an alternative reduced skipping sessions.

Worksheet 21: Structured Check-Ins

Title
Structured Check-Ins

Purpose
You schedule regular times—daily, weekly, or monthly—to assess progress, solve new problems, and adapt the plan as necessary.

The Rationale
Miller and Rollnick (2013) highlight that frequent reviews help clients stay alert to small obstacles, preventing them from escalating. Consistent check-ins show commitment.

Step-by-Step Instructions

1. Decide a frequency that fits the client's pace: e.g., weekly phone call or journaling.
2. Each check-in covers what's been achieved, encountered challenges, and next steps.
3. Keep them relatively short to maintain consistency.
4. Record outcomes or insights for continuity.

Tips for Debriefing

- If they skip a check-in, ask them to reflect on what happened and how they can resume.
- If they find it too frequent, scale back but keep some structure.

Troubleshooting Common Challenges

- If they feel it's too formal, adopt a simpler approach like a 2-minute daily reflection.
- If they forget, add reminders or link the check-in to an existing routine.

Reflection Questions

- Does this frequency feel right for you?
- How might reviewing wins or setbacks regularly help you grow?

Real life application
Steph decided on a weekly Sunday night self-check, summarising tasks done, any issues, and a mini-goal for the coming week. This routine prevented drifting for weeks without progress.

Worksheet 22: Co-Creating Shared Goals

Title
Co-Creating Shared Goals

Purpose
If others are involved (family, partner, or peers), you unify everyone by discussing mutual aims or ways to support each other's individual plans.

The Rationale
Rogers (1957) notes that synergy from supportive relationships can strengthen follow-through. Shared or complementary goals often foster a sense of teamwork.

Step-by-Step Instructions

1. Invite relevant parties to name personal aims.
2. Look for overlaps or supportive connections (e.g., both want to cook healthier dinners).
3. Draft a mini-agreement on how they'll cooperate or hold each other accountable.
4. Revisit it as needed to maintain harmony.

Tips for Debriefing

- Emphasise mutual respect so each person's goal remains valued.
- If serious conflicts appear, help them compromise or find each person's unique role.

Troubleshooting Common Challenges

- If one party is less motivated, explore partial support or separate timelines.
- If tension arises, pivot to a calmer approach or individual planning, then reintroduce collaboration gradually.

Reflection Questions

- Which joint effort are you most excited about?
- How might you resolve any disagreement or difference in pace?

Real life application
Juan and his partner both wanted to lose weight. They agreed to plan a shared weekly meal prep, splitting tasks and cheering each other on, merging their objectives into a supportive routine.

Worksheet 23: Tracking Emotions

Title
Tracking Emotions

Purpose
You add an emotional aspect to the planning system, noting how each step affects mood or stress. This can guide adjustments if certain tasks cause undue strain.

The Rationale
Seligman (2011) states that emotional well-being influences persistence. Observing emotional patterns uncovers if the plan is realistic or needs tweaking for mental health.

Step-by-Step Instructions

1. Alongside your daily or weekly progress log, record feelings about each task (excited, anxious, bored).
2. Identify any task that repeatedly triggers negative emotions.
3. Brainstorm modifications or coping strategies.
4. Encourage positive reinforcement for tasks that enhance mood.

Tips for Debriefing

- Highlight that not all tasks are fun, but persistent strong negatives might signal a mismatch.
- If a task is vital yet drains them, consider pairing it with a small reward.

Troubleshooting Common Challenges

- If they are reluctant to detail emotions, stress it's quick: a one-word or short note.
- If they see no emotional shifts, help them watch for subtler clues like mild frustration or relief.

Reflection Questions

- Which tasks consistently lift your spirits?
- How might you handle tasks that bring negative feelings but are essential?

Real life application

Karim recorded "energised" after a morning run but "tense" before a coding lesson. He realised anxiety about coding meant he needed more tutoring or a simpler approach, fine-tuning the plan for better outcomes.

Worksheet 24: Leveraging Existing Strengths

Title

Leveraging Existing Strengths

Purpose

You return to earlier identified strengths or successes, weaving them into the plan so the client feels more confident and prepared for obstacles.

The Rationale

Bandura (1997) emphasises harnessing personal competencies. Building on strengths can accelerate growth and ward off discouragement.

Step-by-Step Instructions

1. List the strengths discovered in prior worksheets (organisation, persistence, creativity).
2. Match each strength to a step in the plan: "Use creativity to design a fun approach to meal prep."
3. Encourage them to consciously rely on that skill or trait when tackling relevant tasks.
4. Discuss how it feels to use a known ability in new contexts.

Tips for Debriefing

- If they downplay their strengths, recall specific examples from earlier discussions.

- Reinforce that everyone has unique assets that can tip the balance in tough moments.

Troubleshooting Common Challenges

- If they claim no strengths, gently revisit any small achievements or coping strategies they've used successfully.
- If they rely on one strength only, highlight others that can also help.

Reflection Questions

- Which strength do you most want to activate in this plan?
- How can you remind yourself to apply it at the right time?

Real life application
Megan was great at planning social events, so she used that organisational flair to schedule weekly healthy meal menus. Realising she had experience coordinating complex gatherings made planning dinners feel easier.

Worksheet 25: Envisioning Obstacles

Title
Envisioning Obstacles

Purpose
The client mentally walks through each step, predicting real-life bumps in the road. This mental rehearsal fosters readiness and prompts solutions.

The Rationale
Prochaska and DiClemente (1983) remind us that anticipating hurdles can reduce emotional shock. Simulation helps them refine or confirm their plan.

Step-by-Step Instructions

1. Take each action step and have them imagine carrying it out.
2. Ask, "What might go wrong or distract you at this point?"

3. Reflect possible coping tactics or modifications.
4. Integrate these insights into the final plan.

Tips for Debriefing

- Keep the tone constructive. The aim is resilience, not fatalism.
- Praise them for honest self-awareness about potential pitfalls.

Troubleshooting Common Challenges

- If they only see obstacles, balance it by recalling strengths or backups.
- If they feel anxious, reassure them that many obstacles never materialise, but readiness is key.

Reflection Questions

- Which obstacle scenario felt most vivid?
- What quick adjustment could overcome it?

Real life application
Rhys wanted to jog daily but pictured poor weather or oversleeping. His solutions included an indoor workout app and setting two alarms. Knowing these options in advance eased worry.

Worksheet 26: Progress Debrief

Title
Progress Debrief

Purpose
After each milestone, you and the client pause to evaluate what went well, what was tough, and how to evolve the plan for the next phase.

The Rationale
Miller and Rollnick (2013) show that reflective learning cements improvements and corrects course swiftly. Ongoing review keeps the client from repeating errors.

Step-by-Step Instructions

1. When a milestone is reached, hold a short debrief session.
2. Ask: "What succeeded?" "What was harder than expected?" "How can we use this lesson going forward?"
3. Adjust the plan's future steps if needed, incorporating new insights.
4. Celebrate any success or partial success.

Tips for Debriefing

- Encourage specific feedback, not just "it was okay."
- Remind them this is a normal process—fine-tuning ensures final success.

Troubleshooting Common Challenges

- If they're upset by missed targets, highlight partial achievements or problem-solving.
- If they see no improvement, gently discuss if the goal or timeline needs adjusting.

Reflection Questions

- Which new insight do you find most valuable?
- How might you tackle the next step differently based on this debrief?

Real life application
Ava's first milestone was completing a month of mindfulness exercises. She debriefed with her counsellor, realised morning sessions worked better than evening, and updated her schedule accordingly.

Worksheet 27: Guided Problem-Solving

Title
Guided Problem-Solving

Purpose

You apply a structured problem-solving approach to any challenge that arises, ensuring the client systematically finds solutions instead of freezing in frustration.

The Rationale

Beck (2011) notes that a clear process (define, brainstorm, evaluate, decide, follow-up) reduces confusion. It fosters empowerment and calmness under pressure.

Step-by-Step Instructions

1. Identify a current barrier (lack of time, conflict with a friend).
2. Brainstorm solutions—no judgment initially.
3. Weigh pros and cons of each.
4. Select the best option; plan a quick test.
5. Evaluate results and adjust if needed.

Tips for Debriefing

- Encourage them to remain flexible if the first chosen solution doesn't work perfectly.
- Praise thorough thinking—every attempt clarifies next steps.

Troubleshooting Common Challenges

- If they fixate on one idea, prompt them for at least two or three alternatives.
- If they constantly discard all ideas, ask what partial solution might be a small improvement.

Reflection Questions

- Which alternative solution caught your interest most?
- How can you ensure you test it soon?

Real life application

Jacob struggled to find an exercise partner. Through problem-solving, he listed possibilities (joining a local sports group, finding a coworker to walk with, or using an online fitness buddy). He tried the online approach and found it suited his busy schedule.

Worksheet 28: Celebrating Milestones

Title
Celebrating Milestones

Purpose
You formalise how the client will recognise each achievement. Public or private celebrations keep them energised for the next challenge.

The Rationale
Seligman (2011) confirms that positive reinforcement upon reaching specific goals fosters an optimistic mindset. It also deepens satisfaction, making it more likely they continue.

Step-by-Step Instructions

1. Identify key milestones (completing the first week, hitting a certain metric, finishing half the tasks).
2. Assign a specific celebration method (a favourite meal, a social media post, or personal journaling).
3. Ask them to reflect on the emotional payoff of this celebration.
4. Encourage immediate or same-day recognition so the link is strong.

Tips for Debriefing

- If they dislike public announcements, choose a private treat or a reflective ritual.
- Make sure celebrations do not sabotage the goal (like an unhealthy binge if the goal is wellness).

Troubleshooting Common Challenges

- If they never feel achievements are big enough to celebrate, remind them small steps count.
- If they over-celebrate, overshadowing tasks left, encourage balance.

Reflection Questions

- What kind of celebration makes you feel genuinely rewarded?
- Could sharing your success with someone help sustain motivation?

Real life application
Sam hit his first milestone of applying to three jobs in a week. He treated himself to a relaxed day hike, combining exercise with pride in his progress. This reward inspired further applications.

Worksheet 29: Balancing Flexibility and Structure

Title
Balancing Flexibility and Structure

Purpose
You tailor the plan to the client's personal style, deciding how much rigidity they need vs. room for spontaneous changes. This balance increases the chance of consistent engagement.

The Rationale
Rogers (1957) emphasises individuality in therapy. Too much structure can suffocate some, too little can unmoor others. Finding a sweet spot fosters compliance and creativity.

Step-by-Step Instructions

1. Review the plan's current level of detail.
2. Ask them how they prefer to operate: do they thrive on tight schedules or more open guidelines?
3. Adjust specifics, scheduling, or accountability systems to suit that preference.
4. Plan a short trial period to see if this approach fits or needs rebalancing.

Tips for Debriefing

- Acknowledge it's not one-size-fits-all. They can always pivot if one style grows stale.
- Check if anxiety or prior negative experiences with over-control affect their stance.

Troubleshooting Common Challenges

- If they want no structure at all, gently highlight how some minimal plan aids follow-through.
- If they crave excessive detail, ensure they leave a buffer for life's unpredictability.

Reflection Questions

- Do you thrive with precise timelines or prefer broad daily tasks?
- How might adjusting structure reduce stress or avoidance?

Real life application
Ann felt smothered by a rigid hour-by-hour plan but floundered with no plan at all. She tried a compromise: two daily tasks in a morning or afternoon slot, allowing for variation in exact timing.

Worksheet 30: Identifying Mission-Critical Tasks

Title
Identifying Mission-Critical Tasks

Purpose
You highlight tasks so essential that missing them jeopardises the whole plan. Prioritising these ensures progress doesn't stall on optional details.

The Rationale
Miller and Rollnick (2013) mention that some tasks are the linchpins of success. Focusing attention on them guards against drifting in unimportant directions.

Step-by-Step Instructions

1. From the action breakdown, label which tasks are "mission-critical."
2. Discuss why each is indispensable (time-sensitive, high impact, or foundational).
3. Place them at the top of the schedule or plan.
4. If time or energy is limited, ensure these tasks happen first.

Tips for Debriefing

- Urge them to revisit these tasks regularly, verifying they stay on track.
- Affirm that secondary tasks can wait if mission-critical ones face issues.

Troubleshooting Common Challenges

- If they label everything mission-critical, filter further by realistic necessity.
- If they ignore these tasks, revisit the root motivation behind them or adjust the plan.

Reflection Questions

- Which core tasks, if done well, will push everything forward?
- Are you comfortable committing time to these before less vital tasks?

Real life application

In launching his design service, Josh concluded that creating a professional portfolio was mission-critical. He made it top priority, realising other marketing tasks paled in importance if he had nothing polished to show.

Worksheet 31: Reflecting on Past Plans

Title
Reflecting on Past Plans

Purpose
You examine any previous attempts at goal setting, discerning lessons from old missteps or successes. This helps refine current methods.

The Rationale

Beck (2011) emphasises learning from experience. A short retrospective can illuminate pitfalls (like over-ambitious timetables) or strengths (like effective accountability).

Step-by-Step Instructions

1. Ask if they've tried similar plans in the past.
2. Identify what went right and what collapsed.
3. Reflect on how the new plan can incorporate those successes or avoid old errors.
4. Incorporate these insights into the final blueprint.

Tips for Debriefing

- Keep the tone curious rather than blameful.
- Affirm that each "failed" plan was also a source of learning.

Troubleshooting Common Challenges

- If they're embarrassed, empathise that this is normal progress, not condemnation.
- If they downplay old successes, gently remind them of the value in each small win.

Reflection Questions

- Which older strategy might still be useful now?
- How does recalling a past plan's downfall help you avoid repeating it?

Real life application

Elena tried quitting smoking before but set unrealistic timelines. On reflection, she saw a slower taper and stronger social support might work better. The new plan used these lessons, focusing on gradual steps and a buddy system.

Worksheet 32: Setting Boundaries

Title
Setting Boundaries

Purpose
You help the client define boundaries that protect their goal from draining influences—
like excessive demands from others or distracting commitments.

The Rationale
Rogers (1957) notes that setting personal limits guards energy and time, sustaining the
client's primary objective. Without boundaries, external pressures can derail progress.

Step-by-Step Instructions

1. Identify how others or certain habits infringe on goal-related tasks.
2. Decide on a boundary strategy: politely declining extra duties, limiting phone
   usage after a certain hour, etc.
3. Encourage role-play for how they'll communicate these boundaries if needed.
4. Gradually implement them, watching for pushback or adjustments required.

Tips for Debriefing

- Clarify that boundaries aren't selfish; they're essential for healthy self-care.
- Offer phrases they might use if they feel uneasy saying "no."

Troubleshooting Common Challenges

- If they feel guilt or fear about setting boundaries, normalise these emotions.
- If others react poorly, explore ways to reaffirm or renegotiate the boundary
  calmly.

Reflection Questions

- Which boundary feels hardest to enforce?
- How will honouring these limits advance your plan?

Real life application
Brenda decided to limit evening calls from certain friends who often wanted her time
for drama-filled chats. She explained calmly that she needed that hour for study,
feeling more in control of her schedule.

Worksheet 33: Adapting Goals Over Time

Title
Adapting Goals Over Time

Purpose
You ensure the client revisits and, if needed, revises goals as life shifts or new insights arise, preventing them from clinging to out-of-date plans.

The Rationale
Prochaska and DiClemente (1983) emphasise cyclical progression in change. Goals evolve as circumstances do, so adapting keeps them fresh and relevant.

Step-by-Step Instructions

1. Schedule a brief monthly or quarterly review.
2. Ask if the client's circumstances, motivations, or priorities have changed.
3. Tweak the timeline or scope accordingly, confirming the new direction.
4. Record these modifications so the plan always reflects current reality.

Tips for Debriefing

- Encourage them not to see changes as "failing," but as normal life adaptation.
- Keep the main purpose in sight while adjusting sub-goals.

Troubleshooting Common Challenges

- If they view any update as giving up, reframe it as strategic re-evaluation.
- If they never update even when blocked, gently highlight signs that the plan might need a shift.

Reflection Questions

- Has anything happened recently that shifts your goal's priority?
- How might adjusting your plan actually help you move faster now?

393

Real life application

Vikram was half-finished with a professional certification when job demands suddenly grew. Instead of pushing through unmanageable stress, he moved his finish date back by two months, keeping a sustainable pace.

Worksheet 34: Resource Acquisition

Title
Resource Acquisition

Purpose
You plan how the client will gather extra tools, knowledge, or funds needed for success. This ensures they aren't hindered by missing essentials partway in.

The Rationale
Bandura (1997) notes that lacking resources can stall even the best plan. Identifying and securing them early fosters a smoother ride.

Step-by-Step Instructions

1. Ask them: "What do you need but don't currently have?" (skills, equipment, financial support).
2. Brainstorm ways to get each resource—online courses, borrowing from a friend, seeking a small grant.
3. Put these mini-goals into the main plan with approximate dates.
4. Re-check that resource gathering is feasible itself.

Tips for Debriefing

- Emphasise that small resource steps can pave the way for big leaps.
- Celebrate any easy fixes—like library access or free trial memberships.

Troubleshooting Common Challenges

- If they claim they can't afford something, explore lower-cost alternatives or partial solutions.

- If they keep delaying resource steps, see if fear or pride blocks them from seeking help.

Reflection Questions

- Which resource do you see as top priority to secure first?
- Can you think of creative or low-cost ways to fill resource gaps?

Real life application
Tyler realised he needed basic video editing software and knowledge to launch a vlog. He found free online tutorials and used an open-source editor, removing obstacles and boosting his confidence in the plan.

Worksheet 35: Milestone Mapping

Title
Milestone Mapping

Purpose
You and the client sketch a visual or written timeline with clear markers of success, giving them a sense of progress across the journey.

The Rationale
Miller and Rollnick (2013) confirm that seeing incremental checkpoints keeps energy high. It also clarifies that big goals consist of smaller, step-by-step achievements.

Step-by-Step Instructions

1. Draw or list a timeline from today until the intended completion date.
2. Insert milestones—like "Complete research," "Hit 50% of target," or "Finish final test."
3. Decide approximate time intervals for each marker.
4. Encourage them to cross off or circle each milestone as it's met.

Tips for Debriefing

- Keep the number of milestones reasonable so it's not just a clutter of deadlines.
- Visual reminders can be posted on a board or phone wallpaper.

Troubleshooting Common Challenges

- If they're anxious about deadlines, keep them flexible or small.
- If they want open-ended timing, compromise with a rough range.

Reflection Questions

- Which milestone are you looking forward to the most?
- How will you celebrate when you reach each marker?

Real life application
Natalie mapped a 4-month plan for her design portfolio, with monthly markers: first for concept sketches, second for drafting, third for final polish. Checking each off kept her excited and aware of progress.

Worksheet 36: Reflective Journaling on Setbacks

Title
Reflective Journaling on Setbacks

Purpose
You prepare a framework for how clients note down and learn from unexpected mishaps, turning them into stepping stones rather than reasons to quit.

The Rationale
Seligman (2011) notes that resilience often depends on reinterpreting setbacks as lessons. Writing about them can reduce negative emotion and highlight solutions.

Step-by-Step Instructions

1. Have them keep a separate journal section for any day a plan fails or a step is missed.

2. Include: The event, what triggered it, how they felt, what could be improved next time.
3. Review these entries in sessions or personal reflection.
4. Adapt the plan if a pattern emerges.

Tips for Debriefing

- Emphasise focusing on solutions, not self-blame.
- If repeated setbacks occur, treat them as data, investigating deeper or changing approach.

Troubleshooting Common Challenges

- If they find journaling tedious, propose a short bullet format.
- If they sink into shame, remind them this is about progress, not perfection.

Reflection Questions

- Did noticing triggers or feelings around the setback reveal a new approach?
- How might you handle a similar situation differently next time?

Real life application
Leo failed to jog because of late-night gaming. In his setback entry, he saw a pattern: gaming until midnight left him tired. He changed to an earlier gaming cut-off, helping him wake for morning runs.

Worksheet 37: Sharing the Vision

Title
Sharing the Vision

Purpose
You encourage the client to openly discuss their goals with trusted friends, family, or colleagues. This can strengthen commitment through social support or mild positive pressure.

The Rationale

Rogers (1957) believes that sharing can foster a sense of reality for intangible aims. Verbalising them in front of a supportive audience can boost accountability and pride.

Step-by-Step Instructions

1. Identify who might be supportive or helpful listeners.
2. Plan how to present the goal: a concise explanation, the "why," plus ways they can cheer or help.
3. Optionally, set a date or event to share the vision (family dinner, group chat).
4. Reflect on the experience and any feedback or encouragement gained.

Tips for Debriefing

- Stress that public declarations often elevate seriousness.
- If they fear judgment, pick only truly supportive individuals.

Troubleshooting Common Challenges

- If they're extremely private, propose a smaller circle or a single confidant.
- If negativity arises from others, reaffirm that it's their personal mission, not others' to undermine.

Reflection Questions

- Who is the one person you feel most comfortable telling first?
- How might sharing shift your sense of motivation?

Real life application

Chloe mentioned her plan to learn sign language to her best friend. Getting enthusiastic support and regular check-ins from that friend made her practise consistently, feeling more engaged.

Worksheet 38: Accountability Buddy Worksheet

Title
Accountability Buddy Worksheet

Purpose
You formalise how the client and a chosen partner will interact, from frequency of updates to the exact form of encouragement or feedback.

The Rationale
Prochaska and DiClemente (1983) highlight that collaborative methods can sustain progress. Clear guidelines for buddy interactions avoid confusion or slacking.

Step-by-Step Instructions

1. Choose a friend, relative, or colleague willing to help.
2. Agree on how often to check in (messages, calls).
3. Define content of check-ins: quick progress overview, any obstacles, a motivational pep talk.
4. Suggest a small system for praising milestones or offering problem-solving input.

Tips for Debriefing

- Emphasise mutual respect so the buddy doesn't become a nag or critic.
- If the buddy can also share their goals, the dynamic might feel more balanced.

Troubleshooting Common Challenges

- If the buddy is inconsistent, consider another or a group setting.
- If they worry about burdening that person, gauge the buddy's readiness and willingness carefully.

Reflection Questions

- Who can you reliably count on for this role?
- What style of feedback do you want from them?

Real life application
Alan's accountability buddy was a coworker who texted him each Monday about his

weekend study tasks. Having that routine check improved Alan's discipline, and they both traded supportive remarks.

Worksheet 39: Periodic Refocus

Title
Periodic Refocus

Purpose
You integrate a short ritual—monthly or quarterly—where the client re-identifies their top priority, preventing drifting attention as life changes.

The Rationale
Miller and Rollnick (2013) see consistent refocusing as a tool to combat "goal fatigue." Checking alignment with the top aim keeps them from being scattered among lesser tasks.

Step-by-Step Instructions

1. Schedule a simple recurring reminder: "Refocus day."
2. On that day, they list the main goal again, then evaluate if daily tasks still serve it.
3. If they find misalignments, adapt accordingly.
4. Record a quick note on how they'll realign or reaffirm their direction.

Tips for Debriefing

- Emphasise that small realignments can save major course corrections later.
- Suggest they do it on the same date each month for consistency.

Troubleshooting Common Challenges

- If they skip it, ask them to set an alarm or combine it with an existing monthly event (like a bill-paying day).
- If they find no drifting, at least they confirm they're still good to proceed, which can be reassuring.

Reflection Questions

- Do you notice any creeping distractions or minor changes in your ambition?
- How did recasting your goal energise you to keep going?

Real life application

Kylie set the last Friday of each month to revisit her main objective of finishing an art portfolio. Some months, she found no change needed, but in others, she saw new tasks had overshadowed crucial painting time, prompting a course correction.

Worksheet 40: Looking Forward

Title

Looking Forward

Purpose

After one goal is on solid footing, you prompt the client to imagine new possibilities or expansions, cultivating an ongoing growth mindset beyond the current plan.

The Rationale

Bandura (1997) suggests that once a challenge is mastered, continuing to set fresh targets maintains self-efficacy and positive drive. Pausing can lead to stagnation.

Step-by-Step Instructions

1. As the plan nears completion or seems stable, ask them to reflect on what else they'd like to achieve.
2. Encourage brainstorming for the next phase, building on newly gained skills or confidence.
3. If they prefer rest, that's okay, but remind them a new horizon can keep life purposeful.
4. Keep it light: exploring possibilities rather than immediate to-dos.

Tips for Debriefing

- Reassure them they can celebrate current success before jumping into another big venture.
- Stress that curiosity about future growth can sustain motivation.

Troubleshooting Common Challenges

- If they're burnt out, let them enjoy a maintenance period, not forcing quick new goals.
- If they want to leap into multiple big dreams, caution about overextension.

Reflection Questions

- Which new interest or aspiration caught your eye during this journey?
- How might your improved self-belief help you approach that next chapter?

Real life application
Hollie originally aimed to pass her driving test. Once she succeeded, her therapist asked about new aims. She decided to plan a small road trip, then explore future career training, riding her newfound confidence.

These 40 worksheets equip you to design and navigate concrete action plans, turning hopes into tangible, trackable realities. By systematically detailing goals, mapping tasks, scheduling strategies, and building accountability, you ensure steady progress. Meanwhile, supportive tools—like self-care scheduling, environment checks, and built-in flexibility—help maintain energy and avoid burnout. A successful plan is never static; it evolves with the client's growth, triumphs, and changing life circumstances.

Strengthening Commitment

Worksheets here focus on moving a client from ambivalence toward firm readiness. They might involve writing down commitment statements, identifying daily habits that uphold progress, and affirming personal reasons for perseverance. Building resolve reduces the chance of giving up when obstacles appear.

Worksheet 1: Commitment Statement

Title
Commitment Statement

Purpose
You guide your client to create a concise statement declaring what they intend to achieve and why they are determined to do it. This statement crystallises their aspirations and bolsters responsibility.

The Rationale
Miller and Rollnick (2013) suggest that writing a personal pledge enhances motivation. By putting the goal into clear words, clients feel a deeper sense of ownership and seriousness about pursuing it.

Step-by-Step Instructions

1. Encourage them to open a fresh page or note.
2. Ask them to phrase a short promise starting with "I commit to…"
3. Suggest they include a motivation or key value: "I commit to [action] because [reason]."
4. Review it together to confirm it feels authentic and energising.

Tips for Debriefing

- Emphasise that it's their personal vow; the more genuine, the stronger the effect.
- Suggest they display or carry it with them, revisiting it often.

Troubleshooting Common Challenges

- If they struggle to find the right words, help them focus on the simplest expression.
- If they fear overpromising, remind them they can refine it as they learn more.

Reflection Questions

- How do you feel reading your statement aloud?

- Which part of your pledge excites or reassures you?

Real life application
Leila wrote: "I commit to a calmer lifestyle by practising short breathing pauses daily because I value my mental well-being." Reading it each morning sparked motivation to schedule brief, peaceful breaks.

Worksheet 2: Feeling the Benefits

Title
Feeling the Benefits

Purpose
You invite the client to list any positive changes or outcomes they have already experienced, reinforcing that progress is happening and is worth pursuing further.

The Rationale
Bandura (1997) suggests that celebrating even small wins fortifies self-belief. Acknowledging tangible benefits confirms that their new efforts make a real difference.

Step-by-Step Instructions

1. Ask them to recall recent successes—lower stress, improved relationships, small weight loss, etc.
2. Write each benefit in a bulleted list.
3. Prompt them to add a quick note about how it makes them feel.
4. Discuss how these positives link to their broader goal.

Tips for Debriefing

- Encourage them to include both objective results (like fewer cravings) and subjective gains (such as self-pride).
- Affirm the significance of each benefit, no matter how small.

Troubleshooting Common Challenges

- If they struggle to see positives, gently probe for subtle changes (like feeling slightly calmer).
- If they dismiss progress as minor, emphasise that small steps can accumulate into bigger shifts.

Reflection Questions

- Which positive change are you most grateful for right now?
- How does noticing these benefits affect your motivation?

Real life application

After a week of healthier cooking, Greg felt more energised at work and saved money by not buying lunch out. Noting these gains energised him to keep planning nutritious meals.

Worksheet 3: Identifying Early Warning Signs

Title

Identifying Early Warning Signs

Purpose

You support the client in recognising subtle cues that their resolve might be dipping—negative thoughts or patterns—so they can intervene quickly.

The Rationale

Miller and Rollnick (2013) explain that catching early lapses in commitment allows for timely course corrections. Awareness fosters proactive solutions rather than crisis responses.

Step-by-Step Instructions

1. Invite them to recall moments when they felt commitment slip in the past: "What thoughts or feelings showed up?"
2. List these signs (e.g., "I'll do it later," "It's too hard").
3. Tie each sign to a potential action or mindset shift.

4. Encourage them to keep the list handy and practice responding calmly when signs appear.

Tips for Debriefing

- Validate that occasional doubts are normal.
- Suggest they share these signs with a supportive buddy who can nudge them back on track.

Troubleshooting Common Challenges

- If they can't recall warning signs, ask them about times they nearly gave up or relapsed.
- If they feel anxious seeing these patterns, reassure them that forewarned is forearmed.

Reflection Questions

- Which warning sign tends to show up first?
- How can you quickly counteract that sign when it appears?

Real life application
Ravi spotted a recurring sign: whenever he thought "I deserve a break" in a tone of self-pity, he would skip planned study. Now, he checks if it's a healthy break or a sign his motivation is slipping.

Worksheet 4: Barrier-Busting Mindset

Title
Barrier-Busting Mindset

Purpose
You prompt the client to craft quick mental phrases that combat discouragement or typical obstacles, ensuring they have a ready arsenal of supportive self-talk.

The Rationale

Seligman (2011) highlights the value of reframing negative thoughts with practical affirmations. These statements help override defeatist attitudes, thus preserving commitment.

Step-by-Step Instructions

1. Ask them to list their common doubts or obstacles.
2. For each, develop a short phrase: "I've handled bigger challenges," "I can do one small step."
3. Write them on note cards or keep them in a phone memo.
4. Encourage daily reading or repetition to embed these lines in their thinking.

Tips for Debriefing

- Encourage simplicity: one or two lines that feel genuine can be very powerful.
- Revisit and modify if any line becomes stale or no longer resonates.

Troubleshooting Common Challenges

- If they find it cheesy, suggest a more neutral or humorous tone.
- If they revert to negative self-talk, remind them to practice the new lines intentionally.

Reflection Questions

- Which phrase boosts your morale the most?
- Can you imagine using these lines in a tough moment tomorrow?

Real life application

During her gym routine, Alexis repeated, "I've overcome bigger hills than this treadmill." She found it surprisingly effective, pushing her to finish her workouts even on weary days.

Worksheet 5: Celebrating Small Victories

Title
Celebrating Small Victories

Purpose
You help the client to note each minor success, from meeting a mini-goal to resisting a temptation once. This accumulation of wins drives deeper belief in their capacity to continue.

The Rationale
Bandura (1997) stresses that recognition of small steps shapes self-efficacy. Each victory, however modest, cements the notion that progress is real and attainable.

Step-by-Step Instructions

1. Ask them to keep a running log titled "My Small Wins."
2. Whenever they do something aligned with their commitment, record it (e.g., "Skipped late-night snacking").
3. Set aside time weekly to review these victories and reflect on the good feelings they bring.
4. Encourage them to be as detailed or creative as they like, possibly adding stickers or emojis.

Tips for Debriefing

- Praise them for every entry, even if it seems trivial.
- If they forget to log, propose a consistent reminder or pair it with another habit (like bedtime reflection).

Troubleshooting Common Challenges

- If they see these as unimportant, remind them that big journeys rely on tiny steps.
- If they only log major achievements, gently invite them to see everyday triumphs.

Reflection Questions

- Which small win from this week are you proudest of?
- How does reviewing your list influence your motivation?

Real life application

Monica jotted down minor achievements, like drinking an extra glass of water or refusing a second serving. Seeing 10–12 line items each week gave her visible proof of her growth, motivating further effort.

Worksheet 6: Revisiting Personal Values

Title

Revisiting Personal Values

Purpose

You reconnect the client's daily behaviours to their cherished values, ensuring they remain mindful of the deeper purpose behind their change.

The Rationale

Miller and Rollnick (2013) emphasise that alignment with meaningful values fuels commitment more powerfully than superficial motivations. Regular check-ins with personal ethics anchor determination.

Step-by-Step Instructions

1. Ask them to list their top 3–5 values again (family, health, honesty).
2. Describe how their recent actions uphold or reflect these values.
3. If they spot gaps, discuss bridging them with future choices.
4. Encourage them to do this reflection regularly, perhaps weekly.

Tips for Debriefing

- Stress how living in harmony with values often brings satisfaction.
- If they discover inconsistencies, reassure them that noticing is a chance to realign, not a reason to quit.

Troubleshooting Common Challenges

- If they claim their values haven't changed, ask if their priorities or interpretations have shifted.

- If they struggle to see a link, guide them with examples.

Reflection Questions

- Which value currently motivates you the most?
- Have you experienced moments this week that felt deeply aligned with that value?

Real life application
Keiko valued kindness and wanted to reduce her heated arguments at home. Weekly, she reviewed if her communication style mirrored kindness. Over time, she saw fewer conflicts and felt prouder of her behaviour.

Worksheet 7: Accountability Checkpoints

Title
Accountability Checkpoints

Purpose
You create short, scheduled moments where the client or a designated supporter checks progress, reaffirms goals, and addresses concerns. This steadiness maintains the commitment spark.

The Rationale
Prochaska and DiClemente (1983) say that consistent accountability fosters steady momentum. Knowing a check-in is upcoming boosts follow-through on the plan.

Step-by-Step Instructions

1. Decide how often they'd like these checkpoints—weekly, biweekly, or monthly.
2. Define the format: a 10-minute phone call, a text message summary, or an in-person chat.
3. Outline quick topics: progress since last checkpoint, obstacles, next micro-goal.
4. Encourage a positive tone that acknowledges challenges but also celebrates any victories.

Tips for Debriefing

- Suggest that accountability partners be supportive but honest.
- Keep these checkpoints short so they're easy to sustain long term.

Troubleshooting Common Challenges

- If they skip sessions, ask if the schedule is too frequent or if a different method is better.
- If the partner lacks consistency, let the client find an alternative or self-check.

Reflection Questions

- Do you feel more confident knowing someone will check in?
- Which updates matter most to share at each checkpoint?

Real life application
Sonya arranged a weekly 15-minute chat with her cousin, quickly recapping her stress-management goals. That consistent nudge helped her stay mindful amid a busy schedule.

Worksheet 8: Boundaries to Protect Change

Title
Boundaries to Protect Change

Purpose
You guide the client to define clear limits with individuals or environments that can undermine their progress, thus safeguarding the newly forming habits.

The Rationale
Rogers (1957) notes that negative influences can erode confidence. Erecting boundaries lessens the chance of unwanted pressure or sabotaging triggers.

Step-by-Step Instructions

1. Invite them to identify relationships or places that risk derailing them.
2. Decide how they'll handle each one: reduce contact, change conversation topics, or establish strict no-go zones.
3. Write a brief script or plan for communicating these limits if needed.
4. Check in about how they'll reinforce boundaries over time.

Tips for Debriefing

- Validate any unease about confrontation.
- Stress boundaries as self-respect, not hostility toward others.

Troubleshooting Common Challenges

- If they fear backlash, propose gentle, respectful ways to state boundaries.
- If some boundaries are unrealistic (like avoiding a coworker entirely), find partial solutions.

Reflection Questions

- Which boundary will be simplest to enforce?
- How do you expect certain people to react, and how can you stand firm calmly?

Real life application
Joel set a rule: no phone calls after 9 p.m. from friends who often drew him into late-night gaming. He politely explained he needed that time for restful sleep, keeping his promise to better health.

Worksheet 9: Visual Symbol of Commitment

Title
Visual Symbol of Commitment

Purpose
You encourage the client to adopt a small, visible item—like a bracelet, sticky note, or daily reminder on their phone—that serves as a tangible anchor for their goal.

The Rationale

Miller and Rollnick (2013) observe that physical cues can maintain mindfulness. Seeing a symbolic object sparks a moment of re-commitment each time.

Step-by-Step Instructions

1. Let them pick an item that resonates: a ring, a colourful band, a phone wallpaper.
2. Decide on a phrase or image associated with their promise.
3. Place or wear it where it's visible each day.
4. Reflect occasionally on how this reminder influences their actions.

Tips for Debriefing

- If they prefer discreet options, a simple phone lock-screen might suffice.
- Encourage them to refresh or change the item if it stops drawing attention.

Troubleshooting Common Challenges

- If they feel no connection to material objects, try a daily alarm or desktop background.
- If they ignore the item, discuss adjusting it so it's more personal and eye-catching.

Reflection Questions

- Which symbol best reflects your motivation?
- How might a quick glance at it redirect a slipping moment?

Real life application

Terri wore a simple blue wristband with "Balance" inscribed. Each time she glanced at it, she recalled her vow to reduce overwork and stress, pausing to breathe and refocus.

Worksheet 10: Affirming Self-Worth

Title
Affirming Self-Worth

Purpose
You strengthen the client's sense of deserving a better life, emphasising that they are worthy of improvement. Boosting self-esteem can underpin unwavering commitment.

The Rationale
Seligman (2011) points out that feeling valuable encourages consistent effort. Self-belief often correlates with persisting through tough phases.

Step-by-Step Instructions

1. Suggest they write a short sentence or two: "I am worthy of change because…"
2. If they find it hard, remind them of their strengths or previous accomplishments.
3. Encourage daily repetition of this self-affirmation.
4. Discuss how it feels to claim their worth.

Tips for Debriefing

- Affirm that genuine self-compassion can coexist with acknowledging flaws.
- If they're uncomfortable, propose a subtle version, like journalling about daily virtues.

Troubleshooting Common Challenges

- If they strongly resist stating self-worth, gently explore negative self-beliefs or shame.
- If they overdo it in a self-critical environment, help them keep it private until confidence grows.

Reflection Questions

- Which personal strengths remind you that you deserve positive change?
- How did affirming your worth affect your mood?

Real life application
Dara repeated: "I deserve peace and emotional health." Over a few weeks, her

reluctance lessened, and she started noticing fewer self-defeating thoughts when stress arose.

Worksheet 11: Understanding Relapse Potential

Title
Understanding Relapse Potential

Purpose
You normalise that commitment can waver and that returning to old habits is a risk in any change process. Preparing for slip-ups enhances resilience.

The Rationale
Prochaska and DiClemente (1983) highlight that relapse is part of the cyclical nature of change. A realistic outlook fosters acceptance rather than panic when small backsteps occur.

Step-by-Step Instructions

1. Discuss what relapse might look like: skipping a new routine, reverting to old coping styles.
2. Encourage them to list potential triggers for a slump.
3. Plan immediate responses to a slip, focusing on quick self-correction.
4. Emphasise that a slip doesn't erase overall progress.

Tips for Debriefing

- Reassure them that occasional stumbles don't negate growth; learning from mistakes is key.
- If they show fear, frame it as "we want to be ready," not "we expect failure."

Troubleshooting Common Challenges

- If they interpret relapse planning as a sign of weak commitment, remind them it's a protective measure.
- If they feel shame about the possibility, stress the universal nature of missteps.

Reflection Questions

- What triggers might tempt you to revert to old ways?
- How could you quickly bounce back if it happens?

Real life application

Hal dreaded failing again at smoking cessation. By acknowledging a relapse could happen during high-stress events, he created a "call a friend" tactic for meltdown moments, feeling more equipped to remain smoke-free.

Worksheet 12: Refocusing on Strengths

Title
Refocusing on Strengths

Purpose
You help the client remember the abilities or positive traits they bring to the table, so they see themselves as resourceful whenever doubts arise.

The Rationale
Bandura (1997) shows that recognising personal competence stirs motivation. Reminding clients of their resilience or creativity can anchor them in hope instead of fear.

Step-by-Step Instructions

1. Invite them to recall a time they overcame difficulty.
2. Identify which traits or skills helped (e.g., patience, problem-solving).
3. Write those strengths under headings like "What I Bring to My Commitment."
4. Encourage frequent review to combat negative thinking.

Tips for Debriefing

- If the client's self-esteem is low, highlight smaller wins or everyday acts of strength.
- Affirm that each skill is an asset that can fuel continued progress.

Troubleshooting Common Challenges

- If they claim no strengths, gently bring up examples from therapy or personal anecdotes they've shared.
- If they want more advanced strengths, remind them that simpler ones—like being punctual—can still be vital.

Reflection Questions

- Which of your strengths have you seen yourself using most recently?
- How can you apply that trait to current challenges?

Real life application
Megan recalled her resilience in bouncing back after a job loss. She realised that same "never give up" spirit could push her to stick with her new fitness regime, even on days she felt sluggish.

Worksheet 13: Decision-Making Filter

Title
Decision-Making Filter

Purpose
You suggest a simple mental check to ensure everyday choices align with the client's promise—quickly asking if an action supports or sabotages their progress.

The Rationale
Miller and Rollnick (2013) highlight the power of mindful choices. Consistent alignment in small moments strengthens overall commitment more than occasional big gestures.

Step-by-Step Instructions

1. Recommend they adopt a question like "Will this move me closer to or away from my goal?"
2. Practise it with hypothetical scenarios.

3. Encourage them to pause before decisions—whether about spending money, scheduling time, or responding to stress.
4. Reflect how it might reshape daily routines and keep commitment at the forefront.

Tips for Debriefing

- Remind them to be honest—if it's truly neutral or beneficial, proceed; if it undermines the goal, consider an alternative.
- If they skip the filter sometimes, discuss triggers or busyness that made them forget.

Troubleshooting Common Challenges

- If they find it tough to do mentally, propose a note on their phone or fridge as a reminder.
- If they become anxious over every small decision, remind them not all minor choices have major impact—balance reflection with flexibility.

Reflection Questions

- Which everyday decisions would you most like to apply this filter to first?
- How might it feel to systematically choose actions that reinforce your commitment?

Real life application
Ahmed discovered that repeatedly asking, "Does this serve my health goal?" made him opt for water instead of sugary drinks at restaurants. Small daily changes added up to lasting weight management.

Worksheet 14: Ongoing Validation

Title
Ongoing Validation

Purpose
You consistently acknowledge the client's diligence and efforts, reminding them that working toward a better life is meaningful—even when it's challenging.

The Rationale
Rogers (1957) found that supportive affirmation of a person's struggles and perseverance nurtures resilience. Feeling genuinely understood keeps them dedicated.

Step-by-Step Instructions

1. Encourage them to reflect on moments or tasks they handled well, even if they felt uncertain.
2. Ask them to describe what it took—focus, patience, courage.
3. Affirm and validate these qualities, emphasising they're on the right track.
4. Suggest they note these validations to revisit in low-motivation times.

Tips for Debriefing

- Stress that validating themselves daily counters self-doubt.
- Offer consistent positive feedback in sessions, mirroring the process they can do on their own.

Troubleshooting Common Challenges

- If they deflect praise, gently underscore the reality of their achievements.
- If they seek external validation too often, encourage internal self-credit to build self-trust.

Reflection Questions

- What do you most need to hear from yourself or others right now?
- How might acknowledging your effort strengthen your commitment?

Real life application
Yasmin often discounted her progress. Through validation exercises, she gradually embraced compliments from her therapist—then learned to self-validate after completing tough tasks at work.

Worksheet 15: Recording Motivational Quotes

Title
Recording Motivational Quotes

Purpose
You encourage the client to collect or create short, inspiring statements. Reviewing them each day can reignite determination, especially if they resonate on a personal level.

The Rationale
Seligman (2011) notes that concise external prompts—such as quotes—can shift mindset in moments of wavering. Reading them often cements a can-do attitude.

Step-by-Step Instructions

1. Suggest searching for lines that resonate or reflect their goals.
2. Compile them into a small notebook, phone note, or set of cards.
3. Read or recite one each morning, rotating to keep them fresh.
4. Encourage them to note which lines spark the most motivation.

Tips for Debriefing

- If they prefer original words, they can write personal mantras instead.
- Emphasise avoiding quotes that feel forced or clichéd—choose ones that strike a chord.

Troubleshooting Common Challenges

- If they dismiss quotes as corny, propose more grounded statements, maybe from their own journaling.
- If it becomes rote, rotate quotes regularly.

Reflection Questions

- Which quote comforts or energises you most right now?
- How does reading it influence your mindset in tough moments?

Real life application

Carmen found a line by a favourite athlete, "It's the daily practice that shapes the champion." She pinned it near her mirror, reminding her to stay consistent with her physical therapy routine.

Worksheet 16: Time Capsule Technique

Title

Time Capsule Technique

Purpose

You ask the client to write a note or letter describing their current motivation and reasons for change, which they'll open later to recharge commitment.

The Rationale

Miller and Rollnick (2013) mention that revisiting initial hope or determination can reignite passion during slumps. It's like hearing one's own pep talk from an earlier self.

Step-by-Step Instructions

1. Have them draft a short letter explaining their "why" for pursuing this change, plus any immediate excitement or concerns.
2. Seal or save it in a set location—digital or physical.
3. Decide when to open it: after one month, or if motivation wanes.
4. At that time, encourage them to reflect on how far they've come or reconnect with that early spirit.

Tips for Debriefing

- If they feel silly, remind them it's just for themselves, not for public sharing.
- Encourage sincerity—any doubts or hopes can be poured out authentically.

Troubleshooting Common Challenges

- If they fear negative feelings, propose focusing on genuine motivations and a caring tone.
- If they lose the letter or forget, a digital copy can be an alternative.

Reflection Questions

- What main reason do you want your future self to recall?
- How might reading your own voice motivate you when you're down?

Real life application
Theo wrote a letter about his dream to become a calmer parent, detailing his current excitement. Two months in, after a stressful day, rereading it reminded him why he started, renewing his gentle approach with his kids.

Worksheet 17: Involving Loved Ones

Title
Involving Loved Ones

Purpose
You help the client consider sharing their goals or progress with supportive friends or family. External encouragement can reinforce the client's sense of accountability and pride.

The Rationale
Rogers (1957) points out that a positive social environment enhances personal growth. If the client feels comfortable, a close circle's cheering can lift them up.

Step-by-Step Instructions

1. Ask which people might truly back them without judgement.
2. Encourage them to explain the nature of the change and how support can help.
3. Outline what that support might look like: checking in, offering praise, or giving space.
4. Plan a trial conversation or method of sharing (a casual chat, group text).

Tips for Debriefing

- If privacy is a concern, remind them they needn't broadcast to everyone—just a trusted few.
- If tension arises in relationships, consider whether direct involvement is best or if professional help is safer.

Troubleshooting Common Challenges

- If they anticipate negative reactions, brainstorm ways to handle that gracefully.
- If no close allies exist, look into group sessions, online forums, or mentoring.

Reflection Questions

- Who in your life is usually supportive or proud when you improve yourself?
- How could you invite them to be part of this process?

Real life application
Freya told her roommate about her plan to practise guitar daily, giving permission to remind her if she skipped a session. That gentle accountability brightened her practice attitude and kept her from procrastinating.

Worksheet 18: Turning Setbacks into Lessons

Title
Turning Setbacks into Lessons

Purpose
You show the client a systematic way to examine slip-ups, gleaning insights rather than beating themselves up. Each challenge becomes an opportunity to strengthen commitment.

The Rationale
Prochaska and DiClemente (1983) highlight that self-improvement often isn't linear. Learning from slip-ups fosters growth instead of stalling.

Step-by-Step Instructions

1. If a setback happens, have them write: "What exactly occurred?" "What triggered it?" "Which emotion did I feel?"
2. Next, note one lesson or tweak for next time.
3. Summarise how they can integrate that lesson quickly.
4. Frame it as evidence they're building resilience.

Tips for Debriefing

- Remind them not to catastrophise a single error.
- Encourage a calm, curious tone—like a detective rather than a judge.

Troubleshooting Common Challenges

- If they avoid the process out of shame, affirm that self-kindness speeds up recovery from setbacks.
- If the same setback repeats often, consider deeper roots or adjusting the plan more drastically.

Reflection Questions

- Which lesson stands out from your latest slip?
- How might you apply that lesson immediately in a similar scenario?

Real life application

Damien skipped his planned run after staying up late gaming. Reviewing it, he realised the pattern: late nights sabotage mornings. He resolved to log off by 10 p.m. to keep his morning exercise habit intact.

Worksheet 19: Goal Stacking

Title
Goal Stacking

Purpose

You encourage the client to add a fresh mini-goal once they've stabilised or achieved the current one, fostering continuous growth and a sense of forward motion.

The Rationale

Seligman (2011) suggests incremental layering of goals keeps motivation high. Mastering one leads to readiness for the next, boosting confidence and ambition.

Step-by-Step Instructions

1. Identify if they feel comfortable or proficient with their current habit or objective.
2. Ask them to propose a secondary, small challenge that complements or builds on it.
3. Integrate that new mini-goal into the existing plan, ensuring it's manageable.
4. Remind them to keep celebrating old successes while pursuing the new addition.

Tips for Debriefing

- Stress that new goals shouldn't overwhelm—small expansions suffice.
- If they prefer a rest period first, confirm that's acceptable before stacking more goals.

Troubleshooting Common Challenges

- If they overreach with the second goal, scale it back so they don't feel overloaded.
- If they never add new goals, check if they're too comfortable or losing interest.

Reflection Questions

- Is there a modest improvement you'd like to incorporate on top of your current success?
- How might adding this small goal keep your motivation fresh?

Real life application

After establishing a consistent morning walk routine, Esther felt ready to add a mindfulness practice. Stacking these goals created a well-rounded morning ritual, deepening her sense of well-being.

Worksheet 20: Emotional Anchor

Title
Emotional Anchor

Purpose
You help the client pinpoint a strong emotional memory or feeling that symbolises their core reason for change. Recalling it in tough moments can reignite commitment.

The Rationale
Miller and Rollnick (2013) reveal that emotional associations can be powerful motivators. A heartfelt anchor can surpass mere logic when temptations arise.

Step-by-Step Instructions

1. Ask them to think of a time they felt extremely motivated or proud regarding this change.
2. Encourage detailed sense recollection: what they saw, felt, or heard.
3. Suggest they close their eyes and immerse themselves in that memory when doubts surface.
4. Remind them to keep the anchor fresh by revisiting it regularly.

Tips for Debriefing

- If no relevant memory, a hopeful future moment can serve a similar purpose.
- If they experience strong emotions recalling it, proceed gently, offering a moment to process feelings.

Troubleshooting Common Challenges

- If they cannot think of a positive anchor, encourage them to visualise an inspiring future scenario.

- If the memory is overshadowed by painful aspects, find a portion that remains uplifting.

Reflection Questions

- Which emotion in that memory stands out most?
- How might reliving that feeling help you push forward?

Real life application

Rosie anchored herself to the moment her daughter said, "I'm proud of you for quitting smoking." Whenever cravings returned, Rosie revisited that warm, grateful feeling to sustain her resolve.

Worksheet 21: Supportive Self-Talk List

Title

Supportive Self-Talk List

Purpose

You guide the client to collect phrases that encourage or comfort them in low moments. Quick references to these statements can avert negativity and keep them anchored in determination.

The Rationale

Rogers (1957) observed that internal empathy can be cultivated. Having handy self-talk lines fosters a kinder inner dialogue, sustaining motivation through challenges.

Step-by-Step Instructions

1. Brainstorm lines the client finds uplifting or motivating: "I'm stronger than I think," "I deserve happiness."
2. Record them in a place easily accessed—phone notes, a sticky note on their mirror.
3. Prompt them to speak these lines aloud or silently when self-doubt or fatigue hits.
4. Update the list if new statements arise that resonate more deeply.

Tips for Debriefing

- If the client is uncomfortable praising themselves, suggest moderate statements like "I'm making progress."
- Encourage them to spot any immediate shift in mood after repeating a line.

Troubleshooting Common Challenges

- If the client says it feels forced, advise them to adapt the language for authenticity.
- If they forget, consider a daily reminder or pair it with a habit (like pre-meal or pre-bed).

Reflection Questions

- Which self-talk phrase feels most genuine?
- How did repeating it alter your mindset the last time you felt discouraged?

Real life application
Jacob had lines like "This is worth it" and "I'm allowed to learn at my own pace." Whenever tension rose, he'd glance at his phone's notes, recentering himself.

Worksheet 22: Preventing Burnout

Title
Preventing Burnout

Purpose
You explore ways to sustain energy and avoid mental or emotional exhaustion that can sabotage progress. Building a realistic pace ensures steadier commitment.

The Rationale
Prochaska and DiClemente (1983) mention that overexertion without balance often leads to quitting. Balancing rest, play, and effort is key for longevity in change.

Step-by-Step Instructions

1. Check how many hours they devote to goal-related tasks.
2. Ensure they have downtime or playful breaks.
3. Plan small de-stressing routines, like short walks or quick meditations, in the schedule.
4. Encourage them to monitor energy levels weekly to spot potential burnout early.

Tips for Debriefing

- Remind them that a sustainable approach may produce slower but more stable gains.
- Validate that self-care does not reduce seriousness; it prolongs it.

Troubleshooting Common Challenges

- If they pressure themselves to do more, more, more, emphasise the risk of crash.
- If they see no time for rest, co-create micro-breaks or shift less important tasks aside.

Reflection Questions

- How do you feel physically and mentally after a week of your current routine?
- Which simple rest activity can you add to keep balance?

Real life application
Kim nearly wore herself out with daily 2-hour study sessions plus overtime at work. Introducing a relaxing Sunday walk and capping nightly study at 90 minutes allowed her to maintain consistent studying without draining herself.

Worksheet 23: Documenting Success Stories

Title
Documenting Success Stories

Purpose

You encourage the client to research or recall real-life examples of people who overcame similar hurdles. Seeing parallels fosters the belief "I can do it, too."

The Rationale

Bandura (1997) emphasises observational learning: witnessing or reading about relatable achievements boosts self-efficacy. It shrinks the psychological distance between them and success.

Step-by-Step Instructions

1. Prompt them to find 1–3 stories (online videos, articles, or acquaintances) relevant to their goal.
2. Ask them to summarise each story: the person's struggles, breakthroughs, final success.
3. Discuss how these journeys mirror or differ from their own.
4. Note what lessons or techniques they might adopt.

Tips for Debriefing

- If they can't find a perfect match, suggest partial similarities, e.g., same type of challenge but different context.
- Stress that each story is unique, but the spirit of perseverance can inspire.

Troubleshooting Common Challenges

- If the client becomes discouraged (believing the story is too perfect), reassure them that behind every success lies trial and error.
- If they resist external examples, encourage local support groups or personal connections.

Reflection Questions

- Which part of these success stories resonates most with your journey?
- Is there a technique they used you'd like to try?

Real life application

Zara read about a mother of two who returned to university and graduated after

431

juggling childcare. This encouraged Zara to keep up her own coursework, knowing others managed similar or greater obstacles.

Worksheet 24: Daily Reflection Prompt

Title
Daily Reflection Prompt

Purpose
You provide a short question for the client to answer each evening, capturing how they strengthened commitment that day. It keeps them mindful and encourages daily effort.

The Rationale
Miller and Rollnick (2013) point out that consistent reflection yields sustained engagement. Taking a moment to note progress can spark confidence for the next day.

Step-by-Step Instructions

1. Decide a question, e.g., "What did I do today that supports my goal?"
2. Instruct them to jot down a quick bullet or sentence each evening.
3. Invite them to re-read these entries weekly to see patterns.
4. If a day lacked progress, note a reason without shame, planning a comeback move next day.

Tips for Debriefing

- Emphasise that brief daily reflection is more valuable than occasional lengthy journalling.
- If they find it tedious, reduce it to once every two days but keep it regular.

Troubleshooting Common Challenges

- If they skip it, pair reflection with a habit like brushing teeth or setting an alarm.
- If they only focus on negatives, prompt them to find even one small positive.

Reflection Questions

- What changes when you end your day recalling a positive step?
- Did you discover any repeated success or stumbling points this week?

Real life application
Jack wrote "phoned a supportive friend instead of snacking under stress" for Monday's entry. Watching these daily positives accumulate reassured him that he was consistently reinforcing his dedication.

Worksheet 25: Mini-Mindfulness Breaks

Title
Mini-Mindfulness Breaks

Purpose
You show the client how a few calm, grounding breaths or observations can quickly reconnect them to their promise when life chaos tempts them to revert.

The Rationale
Seligman (2011) affirms that brief mindfulness interrupts knee-jerk reactions, letting them realign with their core motivations. It fosters calm clarity in pivotal moments.

Step-by-Step Instructions

1. Teach a simple method: close eyes, inhale for 4 counts, exhale for 4, repeat 3 times.
2. Suggest they do this whenever stress spikes or distractions beckon.
3. Encourage them to recall their commitment statement or "why" after these breaths.
4. Discuss how it feels to pause and recenter.

Tips for Debriefing

- Emphasise that it can be done discreetly, anytime—like at a desk or in a quiet corner.

- If they enjoy it, they might expand to 1–2 minutes or add a mental mantra.

Troubleshooting Common Challenges

- If they resist, citing no time, remind them even 20 seconds can refocus the mind.
- If they find it awkward, propose a simpler version or eyes open, focusing on a single object.

Reflection Questions

- Did pausing for mindfulness today help you notice or correct any drift?
- Where could you see yourself using these breaks more often?

Real life application
Gina set a phone alert for mid-day. At that moment, she paused, did a quick breathing cycle, and reminded herself of her vow to remain assertive rather than passive. She noticed more consistent follow-through on boundary setting.

Worksheet 26: Community Support

Title
Community Support

Purpose
You encourage the client to explore group-based or community resources—online or offline—that echo their goals, offering shared wisdom and solidarity.

The Rationale
Rogers (1957) emphasises that feeling part of a community reduces isolation. Hearing peers' journeys can normalise challenges, further deepening commitment.

Step-by-Step Instructions

1. Discuss local or digital groups that match their goal—weight loss clubs, writing forums, hobby clubs.

2. Suggest they attend a meeting or browse a forum.
3. Ask them to reflect on the sense of belonging or tips gleaned.
4. If helpful, plan regular involvement for continued motivation.

Tips for Debriefing

- If shy, propose lurking or lightly interacting online until comfortable.
- Encourage them to pick supportive atmospheres, avoiding overly critical or negative groups.

Troubleshooting Common Challenges

- If no local group exists, explore national or global online communities.
- If they try one that feels unsupportive, encourage them to find a better fit rather than quitting.

Reflection Questions

- Which community resource do you find most appealing?
- How might group support enhance your confidence or spark new ideas?

Real life application
Eve joined a local meetup of people learning a new language. Sharing struggles and triumphs with peers kept her on track, even when grammar got frustrating.

Worksheet 27: Visual Journey Map

Title
Visual Journey Map

Purpose
You ask the client to illustrate their path, from beginning to objective. Seeing a timeline or simple diagram of achievements can cement pride in how far they've come.

The Rationale

Miller and Rollnick (2013) note that tangible visuals can ground abstract progress in something concrete. A map also clarifies how near or far the goal might be.

Step-by-Step Instructions

1. Provide paper or digital tools for drawing a rough timeline or path.
2. Mark starting point, key achievements, hurdles overcome, and the destination.
3. Encourage creative touches: colours, symbols for each milestone.
4. Use it for ongoing motivation, adding new accomplishments as they occur.

Tips for Debriefing

- If they dislike art, a simple line with bullet points works fine.
- Reflect together on how each milestone reveals their perseverance.

Troubleshooting Common Challenges

- If they see the destination as distant, highlight the many steps already taken.
- If they become upset by a past hurdle, emphasise the fact that they overcame it and kept going.

Reflection Questions

- How does seeing your journey visually alter your sense of progress?
- Which part of the map are you most proud to illustrate?

Real life application

Matthew drew a winding road with small flags marking his completed tasks for building a business. Adding a new flag each month reminded him of achievements that fueled his desire to keep building.

Worksheet 28: Benefiting Others

Title

Benefiting Others

Purpose

You show the client how their personal commitment can influence people around them. Thinking about helping loved ones or community can strengthen resolve.

The Rationale

Bandura (1997) emphasises that altruistic or social motivations amplify drive. Knowing others profit from their success can inspire perseverance.

Step-by-Step Instructions

1. Ask them to identify ways their change might help relatives, friends, or wider society.
2. List concrete positive impacts, e.g. setting a healthy example for children, improving the family's mood.
3. Encourage reflection on how these outcomes align with personal values of caring or contribution.
4. Suggest revisiting this list if internal motivation dips.

Tips for Debriefing

- Emphasise that self-improvement often has ripple effects.
- If they find no direct benefit to others, gently explore small indirect ways or bigger social ramifications.

Troubleshooting Common Challenges

- If they feel they have no close relationships, consider potential future connections or community influences.
- If they rely too heavily on pleasing others, ensure they keep personal reasons central too.

Reflection Questions

- How might your success lift someone else's spirits or well-being?
- Does realising this bigger impact make your goal more meaningful?

Real life application

Marcus noted that reducing his alcohol intake allowed him to be more present with his partner, leading to fewer arguments. Recognising this gave him an extra push whenever cravings arose.

Worksheet 29: Comparing Old vs. New Mindsets

Title
Comparing Old vs. New Mindsets

Purpose
You invite the client to detail how their thinking or attitudes have changed since committing. Seeing this mental evolution can energise them to keep refining their outlook.

The Rationale
Seligman (2011) points out that noticing personal growth fosters self-respect and impetus for further transformation. Observing a shift from old negativity to new determination cements the improvements as real.

Step-by-Step Instructions

1. Split a page into two columns: "My old mindset" and "My new mindset."
2. In the first column, list beliefs or habits of thought prior to or early in this journey.
3. In the second column, add how they now perceive or handle those situations differently.
4. Reflect on the progress made and any remaining areas to refine.

Tips for Debriefing

- Praise each difference as evidence of psychological growth.
- If some old views persist, note them as ongoing challenges.

Troubleshooting Common Challenges

- If they feel they've barely changed, highlight small shifts in language or behaviour.

- If they cling to old negative thoughts, propose focusing on partial improvements or coping strategies.

Reflection Questions

- Which new mindset change are you most proud of?
- How has shifting your perspective eased your daily life?

Real life application

Sarah once believed, "I'm too disorganised to learn new skills." Over time, she replaced it with, "I can learn step by step." This fresh lens freed her to try out training courses with less fear.

Worksheet 30: Encouraging Intrinsic Motivation

Title

Encouraging Intrinsic Motivation

Purpose

You shine a spotlight on the client's internal drives—knowledge, personal growth, health—rather than external incentives, forging deeper and more persistent commitment.

The Rationale

Deci and Ryan (2008) establish that intrinsic motivators outlast rewards or social pressure. Tapping personal curiosity or well-being ensures lasting dedication.

Step-by-Step Instructions

1. Ask them to list reasons for change that come from within (feeling proud, wanting health).
2. Compare these with external motives (peer approval, money, deadlines).
3. Discuss how focusing on intrinsic gains typically yields stronger perseverance.
4. Check in often: "Which internal reward excites you about continuing?"

Tips for Debriefing

- If they rely heavily on external triggers, gently show how personal satisfaction can be more stable.
- Reinforce any spark of joy or self-fulfilment they mention.

Troubleshooting Common Challenges

- If they see no internal drive, explore their deeper needs or identity.
- If external rewards are major, propose blending them with some personal joy to fortify the pursuit.

Reflection Questions

- Which inner reward do you value most—knowledge, self-respect, peace of mind?
- How does emphasising that reward affect your everyday motivation?

Real life application
John discovered that beyond pleasing his family by quitting smoking, he genuinely craved better stamina for hiking. Realising this intrinsic motive, he stayed committed even when family praise waned.

Worksheet 31: Self-Celebration Rituals

Title
Self-Celebration Rituals

Purpose
You encourage a small, personal ceremony whenever the client reaches a milestone, honouring the moment with an uplifting tradition (like playing a favourite song).

The Rationale
Miller and Rollnick (2013) highlight that personal rituals anchor achievements in emotional memory. This spikes satisfaction and anticipation for further success.

Step-by-Step Instructions

1. Brainstorm simple, meaningful rituals—lighting a candle, dancing for a minute, journalling a gratitude note.
2. Tie a specific ritual to each milestone or weekly check-in.
3. Encourage them to stay consistent, treating it as a reward for each forward step.
4. Reflect afterwards on how the ritual's positivity might fuel the next goal segment.

Tips for Debriefing

- Suggest picking rituals that truly spark joy or pride.
- Remind them that even a short 30-second action can be powerful if done wholeheartedly.

Troubleshooting Common Challenges

- If they feel silly, propose a more discreet approach, like quietly breathing in gratitude.
- If they skip rituals due to busyness, keep them extremely brief yet still celebratory.

Reflection Questions

- Which small celebration best resonates with your personality?
- How did it feel to pause and mark the moment?

Real life application
After achieving her weekly study hours, Kate lit a pleasant-smelling candle in her room, closing her eyes for half a minute in thanks. This gentle act made each victory more memorable.

Worksheet 32: Navigating Doubt

Title
Navigating Doubt

Purpose
You equip the client with a structured approach to tackle self-doubt. They'll list reasons they made the decision in the first place, reminding themselves of the initial conviction.

The Rationale
Bandura (1997) underscores that self-doubt often emerges unpredictably. Quickly revisiting original motivations counters negative thinking and reaffirms direction.

Step-by-Step Instructions

1. Have them write doubts they sometimes think: "I'm not sure this is worth it."
2. Next to each, write two lines explaining why they started or the benefits they want.
3. Read these reminders whenever internal skepticism arises.
4. Encourage noticing if doubts lessen or transform upon seeing those reasons anew.

Tips for Debriefing

- Clarify that doubts don't vanish overnight, but consistent reassurance can reduce their power.
- Emphasise honesty about feelings so the approach remains realistic.

Troubleshooting Common Challenges

- If they can't articulate reasons, go back to value-based worksheets or vision statements.
- If doubt is persistent, consider deeper exploration of fear or therapy for underlying issues.

Reflection Questions

- Which reason most strongly counters your doubt?
- How do you feel reading your original motivations?

Real life application
Kevin noted occasional thoughts like "Maybe I don't need this diploma." Reviewing "I

crave better job opportunities and self-growth" swiftly reminded him why he enrolled, keeping him from dropping out mid-term.

Worksheet 33: Stepping into a Mentor Role

Title
Stepping into a Mentor Role

Purpose
You prompt the client to imagine giving advice to someone else facing the same obstacles, which clarifies and deepens their own dedication.

The Rationale
Rogers (1957) found that perspective shifts can crystallise solutions. By adopting a mentor stance, clients may articulate encouragement that also resonates within themselves.

Step-by-Step Instructions

1. Ask them to pretend a friend is in their situation, feeling uncertain.
2. Write or speak the advice they'd share: "Keep going because…"
3. Reflect on how it applies equally to them.
4. Encourage using that "mentor voice" for personal pep talks.

Tips for Debriefing

- Remind them that we often give kinder, wiser counsel to friends than to ourselves.
- If they discover beneficial advice for the friend, underscore how they can adopt it personally.

Troubleshooting Common Challenges

- If they struggle to imagine helping someone, propose a fictional scenario or recall an actual friend who overcame something similar.

- If they feel hypocritical, reassure them that giving advice doesn't demand perfection, just sincerity.

Reflection Questions

- What part of your advice to this imaginary person rings true for you?
- How can adopting a mentor mindset boost your resolve?

Real life application
Melissa wrote a mock letter to a cousin, urging them "Don't quit on tough days; they're just part of the process." Reading it back, she realised it was exactly what she needed to hear herself, reinforcing her vow to push onward.

Worksheet 34: Power Statements

Title
Power Statements

Purpose
You help the client condense their motivation into a short, forceful line or motto that captures their drive and can be recalled instantly for a morale boost.

The Rationale
Miller and Rollnick (2013) identify that a strong personal slogan can rally emotional energy when needed. Crisp words can spark a quick shift from doubt to determination.

Step-by-Step Instructions

1. Discuss qualities the client associates with tenacity: "bravery," "growth," "hope."
2. Craft a statement: "I choose [core theme] over [negative alternative]."
3. Encourage repetition of this phrase at the start of each day or before a challenging task.
4. Revise it if they outgrow the original wording.

Tips for Debriefing

- Suggest they keep it visible on a phone background or desk note.
- Emphasise brevity for easy memorisation.

Troubleshooting Common Challenges

- If they find it corny, adapt the language to their comfort (maybe shorter or more subtle).
- If it stops feeling potent, update it to reflect their evolving perspective.

Reflection Questions

- Which words or phrasing give you a real jolt of motivation?
- How will you integrate your power statement into your daily routine?

Real life application
Miranda repeated "I choose growth over comfort" whenever she hesitated to apply for new roles. This motto reminded her to push past fear, resulting in bolder career steps.

Worksheet 35: Reflecting on Prior Accomplishments

Title
Reflecting on Prior Accomplishments

Purpose
You guide the client to recall other successes in life—whether big or small—to highlight that they can replicate that resilience or determination in their current pursuit.

The Rationale
Bandura (1997) notes that past achievement is a potent predictor of future success. Linking present goals to earlier triumphs instils confidence and continuity.

Step-by-Step Instructions

1. Ask them to list 2–3 times they overcame a challenge (jobs, tests, personal changes).
2. Identify the mindsets, habits, or supports that enabled those wins.

3. Reflect on how they can adapt those same factors to the current goal.
4. Encourage a quick pep note: "I succeeded before when I used [strength], so I can do it again."

Tips for Debriefing

- If they consider old achievements unrelated, draw parallels in coping skills or perseverance.
- Remind them that success in one area can cross into another with the right mindset.

Troubleshooting Common Challenges

- If they only recall failures, gently prompt any scenario where they improved even slightly.
- If they attribute success to luck, show them how their effort or skill played a role.

Reflection Questions

- Which old victory reminds you that you can handle difficulties?
- How might you replicate that success formula now?

Real life application

During therapy, David remembered how he once finished a demanding volunteer project despite limited time. Realising that commitment and time management were key, he applied the same strategies to his new exercise regime.

Worksheet 36: Enlisting Professional Resources

Title
Enlisting Professional Resources

Purpose
You help the client see when expert input—like a dietitian, financial advisor, or

coach—could solidify their commitment by bringing specialised advice or accountability.

The Rationale
Prochaska and DiClemente (1983) show that professional guidance can prevent stalling from lack of expertise. A well-timed referral or consultation can turbocharge progress.

Step-by-Step Instructions

1. Ask if a specific skill gap or area of complexity is slowing them down.
2. Brainstorm which professional roles might fill that gap.
3. Discuss feasibility: time, cost, preferences.
4. If they agree, incorporate seeking or scheduling that help into their action plan.

Tips for Debriefing

- Encourage them to do some research or quick calls first, ensuring a good fit with potential professionals.
- If resources are limited, consider community clinics or free online workshops.

Troubleshooting Common Challenges

- If they hesitate due to pride, normalise that specialists provide objective support, not judgement.
- If finances are tight, explore sliding-scale or pro bono options.

Reflection Questions

- Which professional do you think could offer the most impact?
- How might working with an expert reduce stress or accelerate results?

Real life application
Erin felt lost about nutrition. Seeking a registered dietitian not only refined her eating plan but also boosted her confidence that she was doing it right, reinforcing her broader health goal.

Worksheet 37: Re-Examining Goals

Title
Re-Examining Goals

Purpose
You remind the client that objectives may shift as they develop or as life changes occur. Routinely ensuring goals remain relevant helps them maintain genuine enthusiasm.

The Rationale
Seligman (2011) points out that rigidly clinging to outdated aims can drain motivation. Periodic re-checking ensures alignment with current reality and desires.

Step-by-Step Instructions

1. Encourage them to review each main target monthly or quarterly.
2. Ask, "Do I still want this in the same form? Have my motivations changed?"
3. If yes, revise the goal's specifics. If not, reaffirm it with fresh zeal.
4. Note any new sub-goals that reflect ongoing growth.

Tips for Debriefing

- Affirm that adjusting a goal is not giving up; it's staying dynamic.
- If the goal no longer resonates, discover which direction truly fires them up.

Troubleshooting Common Challenges

- If they see change as failure, reframe it as evolving clarity.
- If they frequently pivot, ensure they're not simply avoiding challenges and help them find the root cause of that restlessness.

Reflection Questions

- Does your goal still excite or inspire you?
- If not, how can you reshape it to feel more meaningful?

Real life application

Adrian originally aimed for 10K steps daily, but after some knee issues, he switched to low-impact swimming. Re-examining the goal let him maintain his fitness path without discomfort, ensuring ongoing commitment.

Worksheet 38: Tracking Emotional Gains

Title
Tracking Emotional Gains

Purpose
You help the client notice shifts in mood or self-confidence as a direct result of staying devoted to their plan. Linking progress to emotional boosts fosters loyalty to the path.

The Rationale
Miller and Rollnick (2013) observe that intangible rewards like better mood often matter more than external results. Recognising these intangible gains locks in a commitment.

Step-by-Step Instructions

1. Encourage them to note whenever they feel calmer, more confident, or prouder after a success.
2. Write each emotional improvement in a quick log: "Date, Action, Emotional Benefit."
3. Reflect weekly on this list, seeing how new habits shape positive feelings.
4. If emotional benefits fade, consider adjusting the plan to keep it fulfilling.

Tips for Debriefing

- Acknowledge that some benefits are subtle—like less overall stress or a sense of accomplishment.
- Encourage them to expand their vocabulary for describing feelings.

Troubleshooting Common Challenges

- If they only track negative emotions, reframe so they see any glimmer of positivity.
- If they can't articulate emotional changes, propose rating mood on a 1–10 scale daily, then linking improvements to actions.

Reflection Questions

- Which emotional benefit surprises you most?
- How do these feelings reinforce your desire to continue?

Real life application
Ben discovered that after consistent journalling, he felt clearer-headed each morning, reducing general anxiety by two points on his personal scale. Seeing that emotional lift spurred him to keep journalling.

Worksheet 39: Gratitude Integration

Title
Gratitude Integration

Purpose
You link commitment to a sense of thankfulness—both for personal capabilities and external support. Gratitude fosters warmth and resilience.

The Rationale
Rogers (1957) emphasises that an appreciative mindset broadens perspective, keeping cynicism or negativity at bay. Gratitude can gently anchor the client's dedication.

Step-by-Step Instructions

1. Ask them to name one thing they appreciate about themselves each day (like patience or creativity).
2. Suggest they also thank one supportive factor, whether a friend's encouragement or a stable job.
3. Encourage them to reflect how gratitude reaffirms their willingness to continue on the path.

4. Pair these reflections with a calm moment (morning or night) to maintain consistency.

Tips for Debriefing

- If they find daily frequency too high, try weekly.
- Encourage detail: "I'm grateful for my determination in finishing that project," not just "I'm grateful for my family."

Troubleshooting Common Challenges

- If they dismiss gratitude as soft or cheesy, connect it to tangible outcomes, like improved mood or stronger relationships.
- If they forget, suggest a phone reminder or journalling habit.

Reflection Questions

- Which aspect of yourself do you rarely appreciate but deserve to?
- How does noticing external support change your outlook on your progress?

Real life application

Before bed, Lina wrote one self-gratitude note like "Thank you, me, for showing up at yoga class." Over a month, she noticed a deeper sense of contentment and a drive to keep honouring that inner positivity.

Worksheet 40: Reaffirming the Journey

Title

Reaffirming the Journey

Purpose

You wrap up each review session or milestone by emphasising that the path of change is ongoing. This final step cements the idea that commitment isn't a one-off pledge but a living process.

The Rationale

Prochaska and DiClemente (1983) present change as cyclical, not a single event. Continual dedication acknowledges ups and downs without losing hope.

Step-by-Step Instructions

1. At the end of a session or a big checkpoint, ask them to repeat a brief statement: "I remain dedicated to my progress; I accept the journey is ongoing."
2. Reflect on how that feels.
3. Encourage them to adopt this perspective rather than seeing success or setback as final.
4. Discuss next steps or upcoming tasks, emphasising the evolving nature of their commitment.

Tips for Debriefing

- Affirm that each day is a fresh chance to honour or renew the commitment.
- Keep the tone optimistic but realistic—this is a purposeful adventure.

Troubleshooting Common Challenges

- If they feel fatigued, reassure them that the path can have restful periods; it's not always intense.
- If they want to see an endpoint, clarify that some goals transform into maintenance, still requiring occasional checks.

Reflection Questions

- How do you feel thinking of your commitment as an ongoing journey rather than a finish line?
- Which next small milestone are you excited to tackle?

Real life application

A final reflection helped Luisa see that even after hitting her target weight, she'd keep monitoring healthy habits. She stated, "I stay devoted to balancing my lifestyle because this isn't just a phase," sustaining her new routines long-term.

Maintaining Momentum and Relapse Prevention

Finally, these worksheets guard against backsliding after initial success. They include methods to watch for early warning signs of lapse, maintain accountability, and adapt strategies when life circumstances change. By nurturing sustainable habits and forward thinking, you support long-term stability and deeper transformation.

Worksheet 1: Maintenance Checklist

Title
Maintenance Checklist

The Purpose
You create a concise list of ongoing actions or habits that support lasting progress. Checking off items regularly can keep you alert to any slip.

The Rationale
Bandura (1997); Miller & Rollnick (2013) state that maintaining new routines requires consistent monitoring. A simple checklist can reduce forgetfulness and stabilise positive changes.

Step-by-Step Instructions

1. List 5–10 behaviours or tasks that uphold your improvements.
2. Write them in a format for daily or weekly review.
3. Tick off each completed item.
4. Revisit the list monthly to see if updates are necessary.

Tips for Debriefing

- Keep it visible—on your phone or a fridge note.
- If tasks feel stale, consider rotating or refining them.

Troubleshooting Common Challenges

- If you ignore the list, pair it with a familiar routine.
- If you see repeated gaps, reflect on any hidden obstacle.

Reflection Questions

- Which task do you find easiest to maintain?
- How does marking completion affect your motivation?

Real life application
Carlos used a weekly maintenance checklist that included "30-minute walk," "drink

water mid-afternoon," and "journal stress levels." Ticking them off gave him a sense of achievement and consistency in day-to-day life.

Worksheet 2: Habit Strengthening

Title
Habit Strengthening

The Purpose
You focus on fortifying the new habits that replaced old, less helpful ones. Deepening these routines ensures they become second nature.

The Rationale
Bandura (1997); Miller & Rollnick (2013) emphasise that consistent repetition cements new behaviour. Strengthening habits reduces the urge to revert to older patterns.

Step-by-Step Instructions

1. Identify the new habit you've adopted (e.g., a morning walk).
2. Decide how frequently you can practise or enhance it (longer duration, extra days).
3. Track progress for at least two weeks to establish momentum.
4. If you skip a day, quickly restart before the lapse grows.

Tips for Debriefing

- Celebrate small improvements in difficulty or frequency.
- If feeling complacent, set a mini-challenge to keep it interesting.

Troubleshooting Common Challenges

- If life disrupts the routine, pivot to a shorter or adapted version.
- If boredom sets in, try variations (different routes or times).

Reflection Questions

- Which small tweak would make this habit even stronger?
- How do you handle days you feel no motivation?

Real life application
Nia replaced late-night TV with a 10-minute meditation. After reinforcing it for two weeks, she added 5 more minutes. Over time, she found the routine more satisfying, reducing her desire to watch TV again.

Worksheet 3: Relapse Risk Factors

Title
Relapse Risk Factors

The Purpose
You identify specific triggers—locations, moods, or situations—that might tempt you back to old behaviours. Recognising them fosters preemptive coping.

The Rationale
Bandura (1997); Miller & Rollnick (2013) note that relapse often springs from overlooked triggers. Pinpointing these risk factors allows targeted responses.

Step-by-Step Instructions

1. Reflect on moments or environments that have previously led to lapses.
2. List each factor (e.g., late-night boredom, certain social circles).
3. Devise one action plan per factor, like avoiding that place or preparing alternative activities.
4. Revisit and refine if new triggers appear.

Tips for Debriefing

- If it's impossible to avoid a trigger, plan a safe exit or supportive buddy.
- Keep the list accessible when going into high-risk scenarios.

Troubleshooting Common Challenges

- If the same factor recurs, recheck your coping method.
- If you feel shame, remind yourself awareness is protective, not condemnation.

Reflection Questions

- Which factor do you find hardest to manage?
- What's one practical coping step for that factor?

Real life application
Lauren discovered parties with free alcohol were a major trigger. She prepared by bringing her own sparkling water or inviting a supportive friend to keep her accountable.

Worksheet 4: Early Warning System

Title
Early Warning System

The Purpose
You notice subtle shifts—like negative self-talk or skipping small tasks—that indicate you might be sliding away from your new, healthier habits. Catching these signs early prevents a full relapse.

The Rationale
Bandura (1997); Miller & Rollnick (2013) highlight that readiness to react to small warning signals heads off bigger slips. Awareness fosters quicker intervention.

Step-by-Step Instructions

1. Look for slight changes in mood, routine, or language that preluded past setbacks.
2. List these signs (e.g., "I start rationalising skipping a workout").
3. Assign a simple, immediate response: calling a friend or revisiting your plan.
4. Practise mindful check-ins daily to spot these subtle cues.

Tips for Debriefing

- If your sign is internal dialogue, challenge it kindly.
- Keep your response steps short and feasible.

Troubleshooting Common Challenges

- If you downplay signals, reflect on the consequences of ignoring them.
- If confusion arises, gather feedback from a supportive person who notices changes in your behaviour.

Reflection Questions

- Which early sign appeared last time you almost relapsed?
- How can you respond more quickly next time?

Real life application

Ethan noticed that skipping his Sunday meal prep was a red flag. Now, if he sees that tendency, he immediately reschedules a time or requests a friend's help, preventing a bigger dietary slide.

Worksheet 5: Reviewing Successes

Title
Reviewing Successes

The Purpose
You frequently look back at your major and minor achievements, reinforcing the real progress you've made and fuelling determination to continue.

The Rationale
Seligman (2011) finds that focusing on wins enhances positivity and resilience. Regular reviews of success confirm your capability to sustain new habits.

Step-by-Step Instructions

1. Take five minutes weekly to recall or list successes—big or small.
2. Note any supportive strategies or strengths used.

3. Celebrate each success by acknowledging your effort and resilience.
4. Decide on one lesson from these triumphs to carry forward.

Tips for Debriefing

- Treat this as a motivating ritual.
- If success seems modest, remember every positive step matters.

Troubleshooting Common Challenges

- If you see few successes, reflect thoroughly; small achievements often go unnoticed.
- If you feel bored, vary how you document them (voice memos or short bullet points).

Reflection Questions

- Which success stands out most in your mind and why?
- How might recognising it keep you on track this week?

Real life application
Abigail used a short Sunday "success reflection." Even on tough weeks, she found a small win—like speaking kindly to herself or finishing a planned workout—recharging her confidence.

Worksheet 6: Stress Management Toolkit

Title
Stress Management Toolkit

The Purpose
You compile an assortment of stress-relief tools—like breathing exercises or journalling. Having multiple options lowers the risk of returning to old coping habits.

The Rationale
Bandura (1997); Miller & Rollnick (2013) show that stress can derail progress if not

handled effectively. A diversified toolkit prevents meltdown moments from leading to relapse.

Step-by-Step Instructions

1. Brainstorm 5–10 methods that calm or refocus you (listening to music, quick walk).
2. Keep a printed or phone-based "toolkit list."
3. When stress flares, pick one method promptly.
4. After using it, note how it affected mood or thoughts.

Tips for Debriefing

- If you find a favourite method, expand that strategy.
- Refresh the toolkit if any method becomes stale.

Troubleshooting Common Challenges

- If you freeze under stress, rehearse a quick step-by-step from the list.
- If certain methods fail at higher stress levels, try layering two techniques (music plus deep breathing).

Reflection Questions

- Which tool do you see yourself using first if tension arises?
- Could you refine or add new ones over time?

Real life application
Feeling anxious, Carla used her "stress toolkit" that included doodling for five minutes and sipping herbal tea. She found it enough to decompress and avoid stress-triggered comfort eating.

Worksheet 7: Mindful Check-Ins

Title
Mindful Check-Ins

The Purpose
You integrate brief moments of awareness—potentially a minute or two—where you scan your thoughts or emotions, staying tuned to any drift from your goals.

The Rationale
Seligman (2011) emphasises that mindful noticing can halt negative spirals. Consistent mental check-ins help you spot small tensions or cravings.

Step-by-Step Instructions

1. Once or twice a day, pause for a minute.
2. Gently ask: "How am I feeling? Where's my mind heading?"
3. If you sense stress or unhelpful urges, label them and take a calmer step (like a breath).
4. Return to your routine with clarity.

Tips for Debriefing

- If the day is hectic, even a 30-second check can help.
- If heavy emotion arises, greet it gently and consider journalling or a coping skill.

Troubleshooting Common Challenges

- If you skip it often, set phone alarms or link it to a daily event (like lunch break).
- If you find it unnerving to face your feelings, remind yourself it's a neutral observation, not a verdict.

Reflection Questions

- Which time of day do you most need a mindful check-in?
- How does naming feelings impact your next action?

Real life application
Gene used a lunch-time alert. At that beep, he closed his eyes, noted tension in his shoulders, took three slow breaths, and reaffirmed his vow to remain patient instead of snapping at coworkers.

Worksheet 8: Flexible Goal Updates

Title
Flexible Goal Updates

The Purpose
You encourage adjusting or upgrading goals once stability is reached. This avoids boredom and keeps you moving forward with fresh challenges.

The Rationale
Miller and Rollnick (2013) highlight the value of evolving objectives. Static goals can lead to stagnation; flexible updates maintain interest and growth.

Step-by-Step Instructions

1. Assess if your current goals are still challenging yet realistic.
2. If tasks now feel too easy, add complexity or a new layer (like increasing running distance).
3. If tasks are overwhelming, scale down or shift the timeline.
4. Set a schedule for monthly or quarterly reviews to see if changes are needed.

Tips for Debriefing

- Listen to your emotional response; excitement is good, dread might signal overreach.
- Keep track of each version of your goals to see how they evolve.

Troubleshooting Common Challenges

- If you resist updates out of fear, note small increments instead of big leaps.
- If the plan is too easy, you risk complacency—aim for a stimulating yet doable step.

Reflection Questions

- Do your goals still feel engaging, or are you on autopilot?

- Which small tweak could renew your enthusiasm?

Real life application
Kai found his daily push-up routine no longer felt challenging. He added a plank hold after each set, making the routine fresh and maintaining motivation to push forward.

Worksheet 9: Accountability Partners

Title
Accountability Partners

The Purpose
You reinforce the idea of consistent support from a friend, mentor, or group, encouraging regular check-ins to sustain motivation and prevent a slide.

The Rationale
Prochaska and DiClemente (1983) show that accountability to another person or community can keep you engaged. Knowing someone cares about your progress often bolsters commitment.

Step-by-Step Instructions

1. Identify one or two reliable people or an online group.
2. Define frequency and method of contact (text, calls, coffee meetups).
3. Decide what to share each time: achievements, struggles, next step.
4. Keep it balanced—both to receive feedback and to celebrate successes.

Tips for Debriefing

- Remind them this partnership fosters positivity, not shame.
- If the partner changes, set new ground rules so each side is comfortable.

Troubleshooting Common Challenges

- If the partner is inconsistent, consider a different person or a structured group.
- If you feel reliant on external validation, also practise self-acknowledgement.

Reflection Questions

- Who is your best choice for honest yet supportive check-ins?
- How might they help you stay on track?

Real life application
Dev met a friend for weekly coffee, each sharing a personal challenge. Their mutual accountability bonded them and reduced excuses, sparking consistent progress.

Worksheet 10: Visual Reminder of Accomplishments

Title
Visual Reminder of Accomplishments

The Purpose
You create or update a visual display—maybe a board with photos or a timeline—to show how far you've come. It serves as a motivational keepsake.

The Rationale
Bandura (1997); Miller & Rollnick (2013) state that physical evidence of success deepens confidence. A glance at your personal collage or chart can re-energise your vow.

Step-by-Step Instructions

1. Gather tokens or pictures that symbolise key milestones (like a certificate or a step-count printout).
2. Arrange them attractively on a board or digital collage.
3. Add short labels or dates highlighting each milestone.
4. Place it in a visible spot—your bedroom or office—for daily inspiration.

Tips for Debriefing

- If it's a private goal, pick a discreet location.
- Encourage refreshing it periodically, adding new achievements or removing outdated items.

Troubleshooting Common Challenges

- If space is an issue, a small folder or a digital slideshow works too.
- If it feels sentimental, stress its role in reinforcing your sense of achievement.

Reflection Questions

- Which item on your display fills you with pride the most?
- How do you think seeing it daily will help during challenging times?

Real life application

Tanya pinned her 5K race bib and a photo from her finish line moment on a small board. Each glance reminded her she could keep accomplishing goals with steady training and belief.

Worksheet 11: Celebrating Milestones Ongoing

Title
Celebrating Milestones Ongoing

The Purpose
You continue to mark each new milestone with an acknowledgement or treat, even long after you've reached initial objectives, maintaining spirit and engagement.

The Rationale
Seligman (2011) confirms that ongoing positive reinforcement keeps momentum alive. Regular celebrations show that the journey never stops being rewarding.

Step-by-Step Instructions

1. Decide the intervals for celebration—maybe every month or upon hitting smaller sub-goals.
2. Pick a consistent method of recognition, like a small reward or a personal note of thanks.
3. Share the event with a supportive person if you'd like external cheer.
4. Keep noticing how these repeated celebrations sustain your drive.

Tips for Debriefing

- If it becomes routine, add variety: unique rewards or different celebration styles.
- Combine reflection ("What did I learn?") with each mini-celebration.

Troubleshooting Common Challenges

- If you feel you have no new milestone, create micro-ones (like 30 days of habit consistency).
- If budget is tight, pick free or low-cost treats (a scenic walk, a homemade dessert).

Reflection Questions

- Which kind of celebration do you look forward to most?
- How has celebrating smaller wins changed your attitude?

Real life application

Jorge initially only planned a big celebration for achieving his final weight goal. He shifted to monthly mini-fetes, like a new healthy recipe session, to keep each step gratifying and sustain motivation.

Worksheet 12: Self-Compassion During Slips

Title

Self-Compassion During Slips

The Purpose

You teach a kinder internal voice for the moments you falter, reducing shame and turning stumbles into learning instead of spirals.

The Rationale

Rogers (1957) indicates that self-critical mindsets often fuel bigger setbacks. Gentle acceptance fosters resilience and the ability to bounce back quickly.

Step-by-Step Instructions

1. List common negative phrases you tell yourself after a slip.
2. Transform each into a gentle statement (e.g., "I messed up, but I can try again tomorrow.").
3. Read these kind statements whenever guilt arises.
4. Notice how it shifts your emotional response to setbacks.

Tips for Debriefing

- Remind yourself that mistakes happen to everyone.
- If self-blame is strong, imagine how you'd comfort a friend in a similar situation.

Troubleshooting Common Challenges

- If you find it hard to be kind to yourself, practise writing or speaking these statements daily.
- If shame persists, consider deeper therapy for longstanding self-esteem issues.

Reflection Questions

- Which new self-compassion line resonates most?
- How might treating yourself kindly accelerate your return to good habits?

Real life application
Joe missed a key step in his routine and instantly felt worthless. Employing a gentler approach—"One mistake doesn't erase my progress"—he resumed his plan the next day without wallowing in guilt.

Worksheet 13: Stress-Busting Strategies

Title
Stress-Busting Strategies

The Purpose
You expand your range of methods to diffuse tension or anxiety so these emotions don't undermine your newfound habits.

The Rationale
Bandura (1997); Miller & Rollnick (2013) suggest that stress is a major relapse trigger. Equipping yourself with multiple coping ideas builds emotional stability.

Step-by-Step Instructions

1. Brainstorm stress-relieving activities—like dancing, journalling, humour, or short naps.
2. Try each for a few minutes daily or whenever tension spikes.
3. Evaluate which approaches yield the best results.
4. Keep the strongest options as your "go-to moves" in high-pressure moments.

Tips for Debriefing

- Switch up strategies so none become stale.
- Use them proactively, not just after stress peaks.

Troubleshooting Common Challenges

- If time is short, pick quick methods (e.g., 30-second stretches).
- If you can't find any relief, consider professional input or group support.

Reflection Questions

- Which new stress-buster surprised you by working well?
- How might you incorporate it into daily routines?

Real life application
Mia discovered that trying a 2-minute "laugh break"—watching a quick funny clip—snapped her out of stressful moods. That shift kept her from stress-eating in the afternoons.

Worksheet 14: Community Engagement

Title
Community Engagement

The Purpose
You stay connected with supportive networks or local gatherings that echo your new habits, enhancing motivation through shared experiences and accountability.

The Rationale
Rogers (1957) emphasises the potency of belonging. Being part of a positive community can help maintain changes because people reinforce each other.

Step-by-Step Instructions

1. Identify a relevant group (exercise clubs, online forums).
2. Commit to attending or posting regularly, building rapport.
3. Share updates or tips, receiving others' input.
4. Evaluate monthly if the community remains beneficial or if you need a different group.

Tips for Debriefing

- If the environment changes or becomes less supportive, it's acceptable to find another.
- Encourage consistent engagement to form real connections.

Troubleshooting Common Challenges

- If you feel shy, start small—like reading others' posts, commenting kindly.
- If negativity arises, counterbalance by focusing on encouraging voices or leaving toxic spaces.

Reflection Questions

- How does hearing others' journeys encourage or strengthen your resolve?
- Which community interaction has most boosted your morale?

Real life application
Omar joined a local hiking group. Their shared updates and success photos reminded him of his own trekking goals, prompting him to continue weekend hikes even during busier times.

Worksheet 15: Visualizing Potential Challenges

Title
Visualizing Potential Challenges

The Purpose
You practice mental scenarios of how you'll uphold your new habits during stressful events—holidays, social gatherings, or unexpected life issues.

The Rationale
Seligman (2011) found that mental rehearsal of tricky situations bolsters confidence. Anticipating how you'll respond reduces shock or panic on the actual day.

Step-by-Step Instructions

1. List upcoming special occasions or typical crisis points.
2. Visualise stepping into each scenario with your strong, resilient approach.
3. Picture how you handle potential temptations or stressors, calmly and effectively.
4. After each mental run-through, note any small tweak you might want in real life.

Tips for Debriefing

- Stress that positive yet realistic imagery readies you, not guaranteeing perfection.
- Keep each visual session short to retain clarity.

Troubleshooting Common Challenges

- If the negative outcome overshadows, try redoing it with a successful ending.

- If you avoid this exercise, explore if underlying anxiety can be eased first.

Reflection Questions

- Which event are you most worried about, and how did you handle it mentally?
- Did visual success calm your nerves?

Real life application
Lana prepared for an office party by mentally rehearsing politely declining multiple alcoholic drinks. She imagined enjoying conversations with sparkling water in hand, feeling confident she could stick to her plan.

Worksheet 16: Rewarding Consistency

Title
Rewarding Consistency

The Purpose
You encourage awarding yourself not just for big milestones, but for maintaining day-to-day steadiness in your new routines. This helps stave off complacency.

The Rationale
Bandura (1997); Miller & Rollnick (2013) emphasise consistent effort as the backbone of lasting change. Rewards for ongoing practice keep the flame burning.

Step-by-Step Instructions

1. Determine what consistency means to you (completing your habit 5 days weekly, journalling daily).
2. Choose a modest treat or recognition—like a monthly coffee date or new book.
3. Keep track of each streak or consistent run.
4. Celebrate only upon verifying you stayed steady for the designated period.

Tips for Debriefing

- If large rewards lead to overspending, use simple or free treats.

- Celebrate consistency, not necessarily dramatic leaps in performance.

Troubleshooting Common Challenges

- If you slip mid-streak, accept it kindly and resume counting anew.
- If the streak concept feels stressful, emphasise a short timeframe to keep it manageable.

Reflection Questions

- How many consecutive days or weeks would feel like a genuine success?
- Which reward aligns with your personal interests or joys?

Real life application

Mara gave herself a star on the calendar each day she stuck to her meal plan. After 14 consecutive stars, she indulged in a new puzzle game. This routine made her less likely to skip a day.

Worksheet 17: Maintaining Reflective Practice

Title

Maintaining Reflective Practice

The Purpose

You keep using motivational interviewing (MI) techniques on yourself—posing open-ended questions, reflecting on feelings—to remain self-aware and avert drift.

The Rationale

Miller and Rollnick (2013) highlight the ongoing power of MI skills. Applying them personally fosters introspection and agile responses to challenges.

Step-by-Step Instructions

1. Set aside a quiet moment weekly.
2. Ask yourself open-ended questions: "How do I feel about my progress?" "Which improvements matter most now?"

3. Reflect out loud or on paper.
4. Note insights or self-discoveries, adjusting your approach if needed.

Tips for Debriefing

- If you find self-questioning awkward, imagine you're giving feedback to a friend.
- Keep the tone gentle, emphasising curiosity, not judgement.

Troubleshooting Common Challenges

- If you skip sessions, pair it with a stable routine (like Sunday evenings).
- If you become too critical, recall self-compassion and reframe your approach.

Reflection Questions

- Which question reveals the most about your current mindset?
- How might you deepen your next reflective session?

Real life application
While journalling, Ben used MI-style queries on himself, such as "What obstacles might surface this week, and how do I feel about handling them?" This introspective habit sharpened his resilience.

Worksheet 18: Detecting Complacency

Title
Detecting Complacency

The Purpose
You guard against growing lax or feeling "I've done enough," which might silently unravel progress. Recognising complacency early re-energises your efforts.

The Rationale
Prochaska and DiClemente (1983) show that overconfidence can breed relapse.

Consistent vigilance ensures ongoing improvement rather than settling for partial success.

Step-by-Step Instructions

1. Ask how you'd know if you're coasting—maybe skipping check-ins or ignoring minor slip-ups.
2. Note these signs under "Complacency Alerts."
3. Plan small, fresh challenges or check-ins when you see those signs.
4. Revisit often to ensure you're still pushing for growth, not just settling.

Tips for Debriefing

- Keep it balanced; you don't want perpetual stress. But moderate challenges sustain interest.
- Applaud your current stability yet remain open to further refinement.

Troubleshooting Common Challenges

- If you resist pushing forward because life is calm, reflect on your bigger vision.
- If you push too hard, risking burnout, step back and find a middle ground.

Reflection Questions

- Which complacency sign do you suspect might appear first?
- How will you break that inertia swiftly?

Real life application
Abdul reached his initial weight goal but noticed skipping weigh-ins. Recognising possible complacency, he decided to try a new exercise class each month, keeping fitness goals fresh and dynamic.

Worksheet 19: Regular Progress Audits

Title
Regular Progress Audits

The Purpose
You schedule structured reviews—monthly or quarterly—where you examine your metrics, reflect on achievements, and refine the plan as needed.

The Rationale
Seligman (2011) reminds us that progress can stall if unmonitored. Systematic audits reveal small regressions or new strengths, guiding timely adjustments.

Step-by-Step Instructions

1. Mark an "audit day" in your calendar each month or quarter.
2. Assess your key metrics (like a habit tracker or mood log).
3. Ask: "Am I advancing, plateauing, or sliding?"
4. If sliding, decide on corrective steps; if plateauing, inject new goals or variety.

Tips for Debriefing

- If data is limited, keep a simple weekly record to consult.
- If the idea feels formal, keep the audit short: a 10-minute mindful review.

Troubleshooting Common Challenges

- If you dread these audits, remind yourself it's a supportive, not punitive measure.
- If you skip them, pair with a favourite ritual like a good cup of tea.

Reflection Questions

- Did this audit reveal any surprises?
- Which small tweak can you make for the upcoming cycle?

Real life application
Laura set a monthly date to check her budget and exercise logs. She spotted an uptick in stress-eating around paydays, adjusting her meal plan accordingly, preventing bigger issues down the road.

Worksheet 20: Mindset Shifts

Title
Mindset Shifts

The Purpose
You highlight mental transformations that protect against relapse: adopting more optimism, flexibility, or self-compassion. Maintaining these new ways of thinking defends your progress.

The Rationale
Miller and Rollnick (2013) underscore that enduring change often involves a deeper shift in perspective. Not just new habits but also a new outlook.

Step-by-Step Instructions

1. Identify a mindset improvement—like being more solution-focused instead of defeatist.
2. List actions or reminders that reinforce this shift (e.g., daily gratitude statements).
3. Reassess monthly if the mindset stays strong or needs refreshment.
4. If old negativity creeps in, revert to exercises fostering positivity and patience.

Tips for Debriefing

- Affirm that mental habits can be as crucial as physical routines.
- If a shift feels shaky, incorporate supportive journalling or discuss it with a friend.

Troubleshooting Common Challenges

- If you only see minimal changes, note small steps matter.
- If negativity resurfaces severely, you may need deeper strategies or professional therapy.

Reflection Questions

- Which new mindset do you find most protective against backsliding?

- How do you plan to keep that mindset alive daily?

Real life application

Kari replaced her old "I can't handle stress" approach with "I can always try one small coping step." This positive reframe helped her remain calm instead of reverting to emotional eating.

Worksheet 21: Planning for Plateaus

Title
Planning for Plateaus

The Purpose
You accept that sometimes progress stalls or results slow. Setting a plan for these plateaus helps you keep faith and avoid giving up when momentum dips.

The Rationale
Bandura (1997); Miller & Rollnick (2013) show that plateaus are normal in personal change. Recognising them as part of the journey prevents negative overreaction.

Step-by-Step Instructions

1. Note signs of a plateau: reduced measurable improvement, or boredom.
2. Brainstorm mini-challenges or new angles to re-spark interest.
3. If frustration grows, remind yourself this is typical, not failure.
4. Keep small data logs to see if the plateau is temporary or needs a significant tweak.

Tips for Debriefing

- Emphasise patience: plateaus can break if you remain consistent.
- If bored, add variety or consult a mentor for fresh approaches.

Troubleshooting Common Challenges

- If you see zero progress, check if the goal is too narrow or needs refreshing.

- If you get discouraged, remember earlier successes and reaffirm your bigger purpose.

Reflection Questions

- Has there been a moment before where you plateaued yet overcame it?
- Which small experiment could jolt you out of a plateau?

Real life application
Harvey's weight loss stalled for three weeks, testing his resolve. Instead of quitting, he tried new workout intervals and tracked protein intake, soon noticing progress resumed.

Worksheet 22: Expanding the Circle of Support

Title
Expanding the Circle of Support

The Purpose
You consider if adding fresh faces—extended family, coworkers, online friends—could provide additional motivation, accountability, or resources.

The Rationale
Rogers (1957) highlights the strength derived from multiple supportive relationships. Spreading your network broadens encouragement and real-time assistance.

Step-by-Step Instructions

1. List people or groups not yet involved but who might be open to helping.
2. Decide how to introduce them to your journey (casual chat, formal request).
3. Clarify what kind of support you want—advice, check-ins, or moral backup.
4. Gently invite them, respecting their time and comfort level.

Tips for Debriefing

- Stress that more supporters can lighten pressure on a single accountability buddy.
- If you're private, pick individuals you trust deeply or focus on a small group.

Troubleshooting Common Challenges

- If some react poorly, move on kindly. Not everyone is suited for supportive roles.
- If you fear judgment, pick friends who've shown acceptance in the past.

Reflection Questions

- Who in your wider network might relish encouraging you?
- How will you define each person's role to avoid confusion?

Real life application

Olivia realised her aunt was a great listener with experience in healthy living. She asked for monthly calls about meal ideas, gaining a fresh perspective and new recipes.

Worksheet 23: Revisiting Values

Title
Revisiting Values

The Purpose
You reconnect to the core principles or beliefs that motivated your changes, keeping them front-of-mind as you face daily choices.

The Rationale
Seligman (2011) underscores that alignment with personal values underpins long-term dedication. Periodic reflection ensures your path remains meaningful.

Step-by-Step Instructions

1. Recall your top values (family, honesty, creativity).
2. Write a quick note on how your recent behaviour matches each value.

3. If any mismatch appears, plan an adjustment.
4. Repeat monthly to maintain clarity.

Tips for Debriefing

- If values shift, update your list so it stays authentic.
- Notice how fulfilling it is to see your life's direction mirrored in daily actions.

Troubleshooting Common Challenges

- If you find no alignment, revisit your goals to better reflect your real values.
- If you're unsure about personal values, do a short values-clarification exercise.

Reflection Questions

- Which value feels most nourishing to uphold lately?
- How has living by that value improved your self-view?

Real life application
Ben kept a monthly note aligning his volunteering and healthy routines with his value of compassion. Realising how consistent he'd become motivated him to continue volunteering and even mentor others.

Worksheet 24: Checklist for Crisis

Title
Checklist for Crisis

The Purpose
You prepare a brief set of steps to follow if a major challenge—emotional crisis, family emergency—threatens your new habits. Immediate guidance can avert a downward spiral.

The Rationale
Prochaska and DiClemente (1983) mention crisis moments as critical times for relapse. A pre-made checklist reduces panic decisions and preserves stability.

Step-by-Step Instructions

1. Brainstorm worst-case or highly stressful scenarios.
2. For each, note a step-by-step approach (call a specific person, do breathing, remove triggers).
3. Keep the checklist easy to access (phone note, printed card).
4. After the crisis, review how the plan worked, adjusting if needed.

Tips for Debriefing

- If you rarely have crises, see it as insurance: better to be safe.
- Rehearse mentally how you'd use the checklist quickly under pressure.

Troubleshooting Common Challenges

- If you disregard it in an actual crisis, remind yourself to practise short scenarios.
- If the steps prove too broad, refine them into simpler actions.

Reflection Questions

- Which crisis scenario worries you the most?
- How would following your checklist calm or ground you?

Real life application

Ada's father fell ill, and stress soared. Thanks to her crisis checklist, she phoned her supportive cousin, avoided comfort eating, and maintained her journalling routine, preventing a meltdown.

Worksheet 25: Reflecting on Triggers

Title
Reflecting on Triggers

The Purpose
You notice triggers that once threatened your progress may have lost their power. Recognising this growth builds confidence and reduces lingering fear of relapse.

The Rationale
Bandura (1997); Miller & Rollnick (2013) highlight the significance of seeing personal progress in how triggers affect you. Realising diminished impact encourages further success.

Step-by-Step Instructions

1. List triggers from earlier worksheets.
2. Revisit each: does it still provoke the same reaction?
3. If it's now less intense, acknowledge your progress.
4. Update or replace triggers that remain challenging.

Tips for Debriefing

- Celebrating reduced intensity can inspire you to tackle any that remain strong.
- If new triggers emerged, add them to your plan.

Troubleshooting Common Challenges

- If you see no improvement, check if you truly faced those triggers or avoided them.
- If a trigger is mostly resolved, keep minimal vigilance in case it resurfaces under stress.

Reflection Questions

- Which old trigger no longer phases you?
- How did you cultivate that transformation?

Real life application
Caleb once panicked at the smell of cigarettes. Over months of positive coping, he now could handle the scent calmly. Seeing that shift boosted his confidence to remain smoke-free.

Worksheet 26: Shifting Identity

Title

Shifting Identity

The Purpose

You integrate your new behaviours into a sense of who you are—e.g., "I am someone who exercises regularly." This identity shift cements changes as part of your lifestyle.

The Rationale

Seligman (2011) says adopting an identity around healthy practices fosters ongoing dedication. It feels natural rather than forced or temporary.

Step-by-Step Instructions

1. Write an "I am…" statement that fits your new behaviour: "I am a mindful eater."
2. Reflect daily on living up to this identity.
3. When doubts arise, reaffirm that this is your reality, not just a passing phase.
4. Evolve the statement if you expand your goals or discover new aspects.

Tips for Debriefing

- If you sense imposter feelings, highlight the consistent actions you've taken.
- Affirm you can be a "work in progress" and still claim that identity.

Troubleshooting Common Challenges

- If you fear sounding arrogant, focus on sincerity: "I do my best to be…"
- If old identity creeps in, gently counter with evidence of your new routines.

Reflection Questions

- Which traits or daily habits now define this healthier identity?
- How do you handle moments that clash with it?

Real life application

Dina used to say "I'm just lazy." After months of consistent yoga, she rebranded her self-view to "I'm an active person who embraces fitness." Soon, skipping workouts felt out-of-character for her new identity.

Worksheet 27: Emergency Contact Sheet

Title
Emergency Contact Sheet

The Purpose
You list key people or hotlines to contact if urges or crises intensify. Having it easily visible can provide immediate lifeline support.

The Rationale
Rogers (1957) emphasises that in acute distress, quick access to a trusted ally or professional can stop a small lapse from escalating. Being prepared fosters a sense of safety.

Step-by-Step Instructions

1. Write down a few phone numbers: a friend, sponsor, relevant hotline.
2. Keep the sheet on your phone or wallet.
3. Practise calling or texting them in smaller issues to build comfort.
4. If you sense relapse or severe stress, use this resource promptly.

Tips for Debriefing

- Include any crisis helplines if relevant to mental health or addiction.
- Let your contacts know they're on your emergency list, so they expect potential calls.

Troubleshooting Common Challenges

- If you're hesitant to bother others, remind yourself that caring supporters want to help.
- If no personal contacts are reliable, rely on professional hotlines or local support groups.

Reflection Questions

- Who among your circle is most dependable for urgent support?
- How might reaching out in time avert larger problems?

Real life application

Marie pinned a small card in her wallet with a friend's number and a local mental health hotline. One lonely night, she used it, finding immediate comfort and a plan for next steps.

Worksheet 28: Periodic Milestone Cross-Checking

Title

Periodic Milestone Cross-Checking

The Purpose

You compare your current progress with earlier targets, verifying alignment and recognising growth. This solidifies the sense that you're firmly on your intended route.

The Rationale

Miller and Rollnick (2013) note that cross-checking fosters clarity. It reveals if you're surpassing old benchmarks or if changes are needed.

Step-by-Step Instructions

1. Gather your initial goal or milestone list.
2. Evaluate each milestone—did you meet or surpass it, or remain in progress?
3. Note any new highlights surpassing your original plan.
4. Refresh your milestones if you've advanced more quickly or slowly than expected.

Tips for Debriefing

- If you exceed multiple targets, celebrate.
- If some remain undone, decide if they're still relevant or require adjusting.

Troubleshooting Common Challenges

- If your pace is different from the plan, see that as normal. Resist frustration.
- If you forgot certain milestones, reevaluate whether they matter or if your priorities shifted.

Reflection Questions

- Which old milestone is now clearly in your rearview mirror?
- Did any surprising turn of events accelerate or slow progress?

Real life application

Thomas discovered he beat his initial weight goal by an extra five pounds, which thrilled him. Cross-checking also revealed he'd neglected a side goal: daily journalling. He recommitted to that for better emotional tracking.

Worksheet 29: Healthy Habit Checklist

Title
Healthy Habit Checklist

The Purpose
You maintain a short list of crucial healthy habits—sleep hours, balanced meals, short exercise—to guard against a slow decline in self-care routines.

The Rationale
Bandura (1997); Miller & Rollnick (2013) recognise that balanced daily habits anchor broader well-being. A quick checklist ensures you don't let basic self-care slip.

Step-by-Step Instructions

1. Choose 3–5 core habits: e.g., 7+ hours of sleep, fruits/veggies daily, 15 minutes exercise.
2. Keep a tracker for each day or each week.
3. Tick or note how consistently you follow them.
4. If one habit dips, investigate why and plan to restore it quickly.

Tips for Debriefing

- These basics often underpin success in bigger goals.
- Keep the list short to prevent overwhelm.

Troubleshooting Common Challenges

- If you get bored with it, rotate or adapt the list occasionally.
- If one habit always fails, refine it or break it into smaller chunks.

Reflection Questions

- Which habit has the biggest impact on your energy or mood?
- How can you stabilise it during stressful periods?

Real life application

Eva's daily checklist had "sleep by 11 p.m.," "eat two servings of vegetables," and "short walk." After noticing a slump in mood, she saw she was skipping the walk. Getting back on track restored her overall positivity.

Worksheet 30: Flexible Problem-Solving

Title
Flexible Problem-Solving

The Purpose
You normalise adapting solutions when facing new barriers or life changes, reducing rigid approaches and promoting creative resilience.

The Rationale
Prochaska and DiClemente (1983) say fluid thinking stops you from feeling stuck if original strategies fail. Staying flexible is key for longevity in improvements.

Step-by-Step Instructions

1. Recall a hurdle or new challenge.

2. Brainstorm at least three possible ways to address it—no matter how quirky.
3. Pick one or two to try.
4. Evaluate results, refining as you see fit.
5. Reflect on how adaptability strengthens your commitment.

Tips for Debriefing

- Embrace trial and error.
- Keep curiosity alive: sometimes the second or third approach is the winner.

Troubleshooting Common Challenges

- If you cling to the first plan, remind yourself that pivoting is normal, not a sign of failure.
- If fear of the unknown paralyzes you, pick small, safe tests first.

Reflection Questions

- Which alternate solution might surprise you but be worth attempting?
- How does flexible thinking reduce stress?

Real life application
Armand's quiet reading time was disrupted by new roommates. He tried noise-cancelling headphones, but still felt tension. Then he tested reading at a local library—problem solved. That adaptability saved his reading habit.

Worksheet 31: Maintaining Curiosity

Title
Maintaining Curiosity

The Purpose
You stay engaged by viewing your growth journey as an ongoing exploration. Curiosity wards off monotony and welcomes fresh insights about your habits and progress.

The Rationale

Seligman (2011) points out that curiosity fosters continuous learning and enjoyment in self-improvement. Seeing each challenge as an intriguing puzzle sustains motivation.

Step-by-Step Instructions

1. Try a "question of the week," such as "How can I refine my routine?"
2. Investigate answers—reading articles, experimenting with small tweaks.
3. Document any surprising findings in a short note.
4. Incorporate the best ideas into your daily or weekly approach.

Tips for Debriefing

- Keep questions open-ended, fueling your sense of discovery.
- Encourage stepping outside comfort zones to gather fresh perspectives.

Troubleshooting Common Challenges

- If you grow bored, shift to another aspect of your lifestyle or a new question.
- If you avoid questioning, gently remind yourself that seeking novelty helps keep goals alive.

Reflection Questions

- Which question intrigued you most this month?
- How did answering it enhance your routine?

Real life application

Elena picked a weekly curiosity like "What if I rearrange my workspace?" Realising a simpler layout eased her daily tasks, she stayed excited about refining other corners of her life.

Worksheet 32: Sharing Your Journey

Title
Sharing Your Journey

The Purpose
You might publicly or privately discuss lessons learned with others—friends, social media, or a small talk—reinforcing your new identity and encouraging others.

The Rationale
Rogers (1957) emphasises that teaching or sharing deepens your sense of ownership. Telling your story cements progress in your mind while helping others.

Step-by-Step Instructions

1. Decide how open you want to be: a supportive group or a blog post.
2. Share your initial struggles, breakthroughs, and what's kept you on track.
3. Listen to feedback or questions; notice how explaining your success clarifies it for you too.
4. Keep healthy boundaries—only reveal personal details you feel safe sharing.

Tips for Debriefing

- Congratulate yourself if it feels vulnerable; honesty can be empowering.
- If negative responses occur, focus on your positives and maybe find a friendlier audience.

Troubleshooting Common Challenges

- If oversharing anxiety arises, limit the audience or detail.
- If you prefer privacy, consider journalling or anonymous forums.

Reflection Questions

- How did telling your story shift your own perspective on your change?
- Did any supportive feedback surprise or energise you?

Real life application
After achieving better work-life balance, Simone wrote a quick blog post summarising her journey. Comments from readers thanking her for inspiration bolstered her commitment to maintain healthy scheduling.

Worksheet 33: A Final Reflection

Title
A Final Reflection

The Purpose
You articulate how you've changed, what you've learned, and how you'll keep these practices alive moving forward. Summarising the journey strengthens your sense of completion while embracing future evolution.

The Rationale
Prochaska and DiClemente (1983) emphasise that stepping back to see the full picture is crucial. A final reflection anchors the progress and sets the stage for sustained success.

Step-by-Step Instructions

1. Write a short narrative: "Before I started… Now I am…"
2. Mention the biggest lessons you picked up.
3. Note one or two intentions for future growth.
4. Read it to yourself or a confidant, appreciating how far you've come.

Tips for Debriefing

- If it feels emotional, take your time and celebrate each realisation.
- Recognise this reflection as both closure for the structured phase and a gateway to new chapters.

Troubleshooting Common Challenges

- If you feel there's still more to do, emphasise that the journey is ongoing but you can still reflect on achievements.
- If negative thoughts overshadow your reflection, remind yourself of the many worksheets and successes documented.

Reflection Questions

- Which personal change do you treasure most from this journey?

- How do you plan to protect and nurture these gains as life continues?

Real life application
Riley wrote: "I used to dread mornings, relying on sugary snacks to cope. Now, I wake up earlier and start with a brief jog. I've learned consistency and honesty about my feelings are key. I want to keep evolving by exploring new activities each season." This closing reflection sealed her belief in the lasting nature of her progress.

By working through these 40 worksheets, you'll anchor your newfound habits and safeguard against relapses. You'll build robust stress-coping strategies, update goals as life changes, celebrate regular achievements, and keep a vigilant eye on subtle warning signs. Relapse prevention is not about fearing mistakes but embracing your power to adapt, learn, and continually grow. Your journey continues, supported by a blend of readiness, resilience, and renewed confidence in who you are becoming.

Reference

Bandura, A. (1997)

Self-Efficacy: The Exercise of Control. New York: W.H. Freeman.

Beck, J.S. (2011)

Cognitive Behavior Therapy: Basics and Beyond. 2nd edn. New York: The Guilford Press.

Deci, E.L. and Ryan, R.M. (2008)

'Facilitating optimal motivation and psychological well-being across life's domains', *Canadian Psychology*, 49(1), pp. 14–23.

Egan, G. (2013)

The Skilled Helper: A Problem-Management and Opportunity-Development Approach to Helping. 10th edn. Belmont, CA: Brooks/Cole, Cengage Learning.

Gallagher, S. and Vella-Brodrick, D.A. (2008)

'Social support and emotional intelligence as predictors of subjective well-being', *Personality and Individual Differences*, 44(7), pp. 1551–1561.

Hill, C.E. (2010)

Helping Skills: Facilitating Exploration, Insight, and Action. 3rd edn. Washington, DC: American Psychological Association.

Kabat-Zinn, J. (1990)

Full Catastrophe Living: Using the Wisdom of Your Body and Mind to Face Stress, Pain, and Illness. New York: Delacorte.

Lambert, M.J. (2013)

'The efficacy and effectiveness of psychotherapy', in Lambert, M.J. (ed.) *Bergin and Garfield's Handbook of Psychotherapy and Behavior Change.* 6th edn. New York: Wiley, pp. 169–218.

Linehan, M.M. (1993)

Cognitive-Behavioral Treatment of Borderline Personality Disorder. New York: The Guilford Press.

Lockwood, P., Jordan, C.H. and Kunda, Z. (2005)

'Motivation by positive or negative role models: Regulatory focus determines who will best inspire us', *Journal of Personality and Social Psychology*, 89(2), pp. 282–292.

Marlatt, G.A. and Gordon, J.R. (1985)

Relapse Prevention: Maintenance Strategies in the Treatment of Addictive Behaviors. New York: Guilford Press.

Miller, W.R. and Rollnick, S. (2013)

Motivational Interviewing: Helping People Change. 3rd edn. New York: The Guilford Press.

Neff, K.D. (2011)

Self-Compassion: The Proven Power of Being Kind to Yourself. New York: William Morrow.

Pennebaker, J.W. (1997)

Opening Up: The Healing Power of Expressing Emotions. New York: Guilford Press.

Prochaska, J.O. and DiClemente, C.C. (1983)

'Stages and processes of self-change of smoking: Toward an integrative model of change', *Journal of Consulting and Clinical Psychology*, 51(3), pp. 390–395.

Rogers, C.R. (1957)

'The necessary and sufficient conditions of therapeutic personality change', *Journal of Consulting Psychology*, 21(2), pp. 95–103.

Rollnick, S. and Allison, J. (2004)

'Motivational Interviewing', *BMJ*, 328(7445), pp. 1402–1405.

Ryan, R.M. and Deci, E.L. (2000)
'Self-determination theory and the facilitation of intrinsic motivation, social development, and well-being', *American Psychologist*, 55(1), pp. 68–78.

Safran, J.D. and Muran, J.C. (2000)
Negotiating the Therapeutic Alliance: A Relational Treatment Guide. New York: Guilford Press.

Seligman, M.E.P. (2011)
Flourish: A Visionary New Understanding of Happiness and Well-being. New York: Free Press.

Seligman, M.E.P. and Csikszentmihalyi, M. (2000)
'Positive psychology: An introduction', *American Psychologist*, 55(1), pp. 5–14.

Sheldon, K.M. and Kasser, T. (1998)
'Pursuing personal goals: Skills enable progress, but not all progress is beneficial', *Personality and Social Psychology Bulletin*, 24(12), pp. 1319–1331.

Sheldon, K.M. and Lyubomirsky, S. (2006)
'Achieving sustainable gains in happiness: Change your actions, not your circumstances', *Journal of Happiness Studies*, 7(1), pp. 55–86.

Skinner, B.F. (1953)
Science and Human Behavior. New York: Macmillan.

Sue, D.W. and Sue, D. (2012)
Counseling the Culturally Diverse: Theory and Practice. 6th edn. Hoboken, NJ: Wiley.

www.ingramcontent.com/pod-product-compliance
Lightning Source LLC
Chambersburg PA
CBHW080223270326
41926CB00020B/4123